"Use of these so-called 'miracle foods' comes as no surprise to me. My early retirement from dentistry was caused by my being unable to no longer stand for the many necessary hours, due to the sudden developement of severe leg pains from diabetic neuropathy. The surface pain on my legs was so great that I couldn't wear long pants nor could I stand up from a sitting position without help. BREWER'S YEAST and LECITHIN put me back on my feet after a knowledgeable doctor prescribed them over a six-month period. Therefore, one can see why I recommend, to all ages, the nutritional path to good health outlined in this book."

Garth N. Huckins, DDS

Having known Mr. Miller for quite some years, here's how I felt after having had the privilege of reading this manuscript prior to publication.....

"It's not how much nutrition you know that keeps you healthy; it's how much nutrition you practice.....this book guides one along the path to health with very simple formulas for attaining and keeping excellent health."

Kimberly Johnson, B.S.
Human Nutrition and Foods

Cover design, layout and illustrations done by John Jones III.

The following pages, including other illustrations, courtesy and permission of:

Page 14 -- *Tampa Tribune* and King Features Syndicate
Page 26 -- Keats Publishing Co., Inc., New Caanan, CT
Page 41 -- *American Health* Magazine, New York, NY
Pages 60 & 61 -- Mark Miller, Ben Marl Vineyards, Marlboro, NY
Page 66 -- The *News Journal* Co., Wilmington, DE
Pages 55 & 82 -- The *Baltimore Sun*, Baltimore, MD, by staff writers Jonathan Bor and Diana K. Sugg.
Epilogue on Vitamin E, reprinted permission of: University of California at Berkely *Wellness Letter*© *Health Letter Associates, 1993.*

Manufactured in the United States of America

ISBN 1-57502-345-8

Printed in the USA by

Morris Publishing
3212 E. Hwy 30
Kearney, NE 68847
800-650-7888

My Lifetime Tidbits

of

PREVENTIVE

MEDICINE

Fran Miller

Health-Mor Publishers
PO Box 361--Georgetown, DE 19947

Thanks, to those professionals who have given freely of their time in reviewing my writings and given me guidance and invaluable advice during this endeavor.

Dr. E. Mark Johnson and Dr. Elizabeth Burke, practicing physicians who also spent a great deal of their leisure time reading and advising on medical points herein......

Dr. M. J. O'Connell, former area Assistant Superintendent of Schools, Baltimore and currently Assistant Superintendent of Calvert County, MD Public Schools, for his thoughts and assistance, especially in relation to school food programs and the concentration on reduction of fat in lunch programs......

Dr. Larry Bockstahler, Research Biophysicist/ Biochemist for a food-related branch of the United States Government, for his extensive review and guidance......

Mr. Charles Worral of Central Soya, Inc., Ft. Wayne, Ind. for his help in my understanding of the complex composition of lecithin, helping me present it in plain laymen's terms in Chapter Eight....

and

To all the medical researchers who are spending their lives in laboratories working diligently for the betterment of mankind.

Dedicated To:

My Mother from whom I received
my early nutrition.....and.....

My Father who instilled in me a most
productive work ethic.

To my wife for her understanding
through these many months of
being a "computer widow."

To my children, whom I'm proud to
say, have accepted the "gospel of
nutrition" as preached by their father,
and have passed it on to another
generation, our grandchildren.

A special dedication and remembrance to:
JACOBUS RINSE, Ph. D
for having taken time from his busy schedule of research to completely review my manuscript, page by page, advising on many scientific results of previous and on-going research and keeping me from any gross inaccuracies. "Jay," as he was fondly known to me, passed away in 1993, at the age of 93, forty-two years after doctors had given him "just a few years" to live after his heart attack at age 51. I will miss visiting with him and Mrs. Rinse at their beautiful retreat in the woods of Vermont.

It is the author's intention throughout this book to present nutritional facts which will possibly eliminate some form of illness before it strikes —PREVENTIVE MEDICINE. I implore the reader to adopt whatever item which I present herein that applies to your own personal situation, regardless of your age. It could save thousands of dollars in medical bills and future years of pain and anguish, as well as lead to an extended healthier "Golden Years."

PROLOGUE

Several months ago, a prominent east coast newspaper published a letter to the editor which outlined ***totally*** what the author of this book is endeavoring to emphasize throughout--***preventive medicine***. The letter was written by a doctor who was dean of a most prestigious school of public health. The doctor had just returned from an international meeting in Europe where it was stated that recent research had found that providing children with a certain nutrient in their diet, costing ***just a few cents per year,*** would provide protection and prevention of death ***for millions of children throughout the world*** The nutrient wasn't mentioned but perhaps it is one of those mentioned below.

The doctor's letter to the editor was prompted by an announcement that a hospital was about to spend millions of dollars to build a center to ***treat*** cancer patients. He was not critical of these plans, explaining that he felt very little will be accomplished until a program is developed ***(which could begin with diet and nutrition as outlined herein)*** to ***prevent*** cancer in the first place, thereby protecting future generations.

The past practice of medical schools in the United States provide only a few hours study on nutrition, in approximately eight years of study and training, and the author hopes that the present day curriculum has changed to include more on nutrition. In an article published about Japanese medical schools, the routine seemed to be very similar to our own in teaching ***treatment*** of illness and disease instead of ***prevention.***

One doctor used polio as an example of disease conquered and practically eliminated from our hemisphere, but this author notes that polio was not cured by nutrition but was eliminated by the discovery of a very effective vaccine.

A recent newspaper headline......

"NUTRIENT DEFICIENCIES BLAMED FOR HEALTH WOES"

The article stated that about **one billion** people are ill or disabled because they do not eat enough of **three vital nutrients** which would cost only **$1.00 per year for each affected person**, as reported by a World Bank nutritionist. Deficiencies of **Vitamin A, Iodine and Iron** cause blindness, goiter, anemia, retardation and death in **more than one billion people** throughout the world.

Millions of dollars spent on global nutrition are wasted on obscure academic research due to governments opposition to consumer education. A good example is the root of the cassava, a staple food in Africa (we use it as tapioca), but the leaves containing nutrient-packed vitamin A are thrown away!

The simple addition of Iodine to salt (as China is now doing using a $27 million loan from the World Bank) would reduce this deficiency drastically. In Mali, the World Bank funded the addition of Iron to water by having every bucket of water wash over an Iodine pack, which reduced the iodine deficiency **in 500,000 people from 94% to 40% In the past year, at a cost of only 10 cents per person per year!**

We can now understand why the doctor mentioned above had reservations about spending a large outlay for a new cancer center when so much could be accomplished by nutritional education.

The March 1993 issue of the *AARP Bulletin,* a publication of the American Association of Retired Persons, had a full page article on Dr. C. Everett Koop, the former outspoken Surgeon General of the United States. The reader will find Dr. Koop quoted herein from newspaper reports, similar to the AARP interview, advising a more responsive attention to ***preventive medicine*** **by changing one's diet, exercise routine and resisting over-consumption of foods**, all of which affect the risk of coronary heart disease, stroke, diabetes and some types of cancer.

One of Dr. Koop's statements that Americans are **"waddling"** their way to an early grave should cause the casual reader to study what is contained within these pages, adopting whatever seems essential in improving one's health.

TABLE OF CONTENTS

Any dietary recommendations discussed herein should not substitute for the nutritional guidance of your physician. A health professional may be aware of specifics concerning your health which may preclude you from applying the nutritional therapy presented in this guide.

FOREWORD

Everyone thinks they want to write a book, especially when reaching a certain age (usually when older), but most of us never get around to do so. Why? Mostly because of the usual lethargy which comes with age, as well as the fact that to do so takes a definite work schedule after having just completed a lifetime of same. I am probably no different than most people my age, except that I do wish to record happenings and events relative to health during my life which have definitely guided my "way through life." It's been a long and sometimes lonely business life, especially following the collapse of an organization which I had established and nurtured to success, said collapse having been caused by my having taken a partner many years after having seen my father's partnership deteriorate due to the incompatibility of brothers. I should have profited from my father's experience but was too cocky to think the same thing could happen to me.

How I kept my health through all that has transpired through the years is really the prime reason for my putting myself through the necessary routine of working with a word processor, today's method of "putting pen to paper." I hope that some of the health tips relative to ***preventive medicine*** which I have followed through the years will be of help and benefit to anyone reading same, though I am not foolish enough to think that *everybody* who reads this will accept my theories (those I've adopted) as their "gospel of health." Maybe one or two items will benefit you and enable you to have a happier and more healthy life, or, give you a track to run on.

I ask the reader to keep an open mind where I mention any personal dietary practice due to one's own belief, religious or otherwise, for I am endeavoring to report in an unbiased manner what I have obtained from my readings and personal diet through the years. The author has the greatest respect for individuals and groups following any method of moderation in their daily diets. You will discover as you read on that I also believe in moderation, as quoted in the words of King Lemuel, from the Book of Proverbs, Chapter 31-6:

"Give strong drink to him that is ready to perish,
and wine unto those that be heavy of hearts."

TO COLLECT ALL THE DATA HEREIN THE AUTHOR SPENT QUITE A FEW YEARS, AND THE TASK OF "GETTING IT ALL TOGETHER" HAS BEEN OVER A TWO-YEAR PERIOD. THERE HAVE BEEN QUITE A FEW HEALTH ANNOUNCEMENTS RELATIVE TO RESEARCH DURING THIS PERIOD, BUT NONE OF WHICH CHANGE THE BASICS IN DIET AND THE SEARCH TO IMPROVE OUR HEALTH BY ENDEAVORING TO FOLLOW A BASIC DIET OF NON-PROCESSED FOODS, CUTTING DOWN ON FATS AND SODIUM.

CHAPTER ONE

MY LIBRARY OF HEALTH

Though I list a bibliography in the appendix, I confess to having saved through the years material of interest relative to ***preventive medicine***, health and nutrition articles from newspapers, health newsletters, many, many books by authors associated with nutrition, whether they are doctors, chemists, nutritionists or just plain people like myself who have devoted time throughout life endeavoring to devour any item relating to one's health. I am also fortunate in having the use of the excellent Delaware Technical & Community College library while taking courses there as a senior citizen.

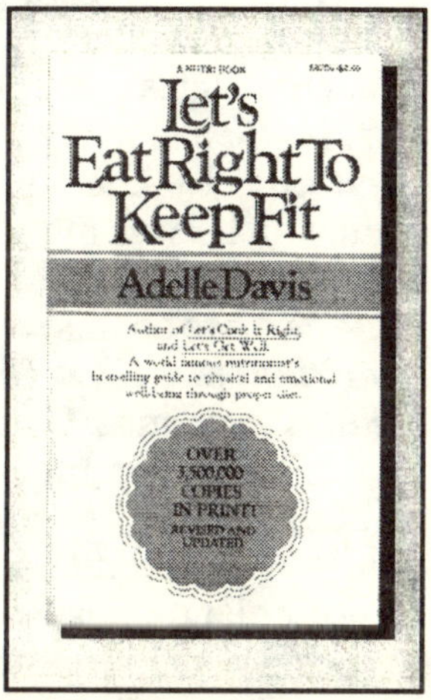

My search for health began with a heart attack—coronary insufficiency—at age 40, brought on by heavy smoking and the stress of every day management of building a sales organization in a very competitive market area. At that time, I was introduced, by my father-in-law (a nut on health!) to the writings of Adelle Davis, who became known as the "Guru of Health Writers." Her basic book, ***Let's Eat Right To Keep Fit***,[1] truly a treatise on ***preventive medicine*** (my copy now pretty well worn out), along with the guidance of a wonderful doctor who had responded at one-AM to my wife's frantic call (they made house calls in those days!), guided me into a new life of organic foods, whole grains and no smoking, from which I have not deviated a great deal these past 35 years.

When all had settled as far as worry and fear were concerned I can remember my doctor advising, "Now perhaps you'll learn how to live and relax." I did, but in the ensuing years I can remember this ex-football player examining me and advising I lose 10 pounds as his gut hung over his belt. My response, "This is the pot calling the kettle black!" His response, "Don't do as I do, do as I say!" I did—he didn't—to the tune of his stroke and heart attack a few years later, brought on by overwork and good living, accompanied by high blood pressure, the end of a brilliant career. Sorrowful! I really missed that guy! When I was just 36 years of age, two small kids and another on the way, I developed ulcers. I had changed companies on a straight commission basis and he knew I was scraping the bottom of the barrel financially, so his treatment was free. Not many of those people left! I sure wish he had practiced ***preventive medicine!***

I will list a bibliography, but, have to mention the afore-mentioned book by Adelle Davis, ***The Whole Grain Cookbook***[2] by Vrest Orton, Vermont Country Store, the excellent ***University of California Wellness Letter***[7] (rated #1 by U.S. News & World Report), ***Eat Better, Live Better,***[3] Reader's Digest, ***Prevention, American Health*** and many other magazines, ***Lecithin***[4] by Carlson Wade (1981), from which I was introduced to the Dr. Rinse breakfast and ***The Rinse Formula,***[5] (more on this later), ***Know Your Nutrition***[6] and ***How To Improve Your Health***, by Linda Clark, all three by Keats Publishing, Inc., plus a shelf-full of books related to ***preventive medicine***, health and diet, including an old New England cook book of healthful recipes. What a treasure I possess for which I am ever thankful as I enjoy my senior years with a wonderful family and enjoying excellent health.

When I speak of "excellent health," it does not mean that a few of the "blessings of old age" have not followed me into my senior years, such as cataracts, slight high blood pressure (high normal says my doctor), a family heritage, sun-damaged skin and a bit of gout. I used to love liver, beef and kidney pie, especially when visiting Bermuda (my English heritage), but have now learned that I can live without them. And, oh yes, a touch of chronic arthritis now and then. However, I learned to try to ignore these little pains and accept them as a re-

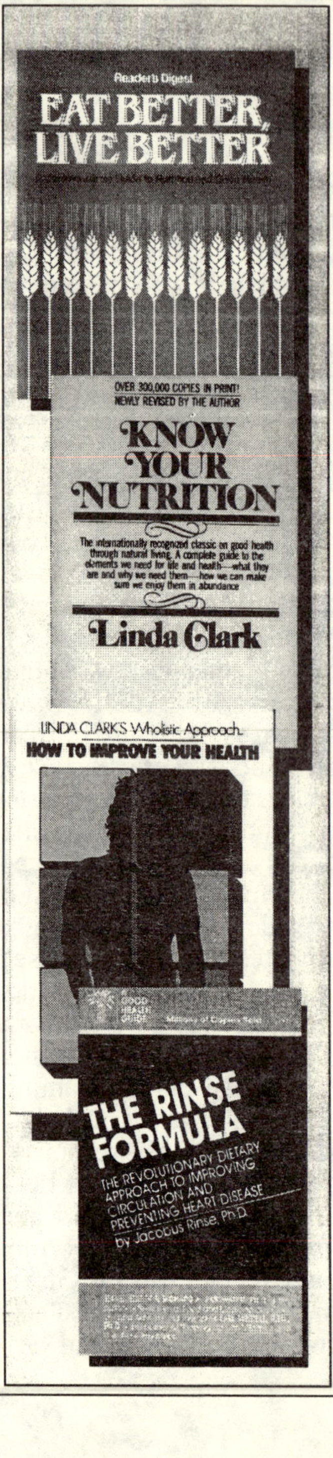

minder that I'm not 36 any more! It's no fun complaining about these aches and pains because young people don't want to hear about them and my peers have their own to be concerned about!

Had we been concerned about the ozone layer and what the sun rays were doing to our skin years ago, perhaps I would not be treating for the neglect towards my skin, which resulted in having treatment 5 years ago for keratosis and potential skin cancer. But, would any of us in youth have listened had we been warned? I doubt it as I watch the young sunbathers of today. Presently, I've also been taking treatment for same at the famous Johns Hopkins University Hospital, Baltimore, MD. They also, along with approximately 100 other publishers, are now producing an excellent health news letter and recently have published the *Johns Hopkins Medical Handbook.* I mentioned the ***University of California Wellness Letter***[7] previously, and it's #1 rating by the *US News & World Report* back in 1987. Having subscribed for a few years, I had saved many issues as a reference. Since that time the group of doctors who edit the *Wellness Letter* have published an excellent book entitled, ***The Wellness Encyclopedia***,[31] covering (their title), "The Comprehensive Family Resource for Safeguarding Health and ***Preventing*** Illness," which I would recommend to any person interested in doing just that. It is most comprehensive but is not a do-it-yourself medical text book.

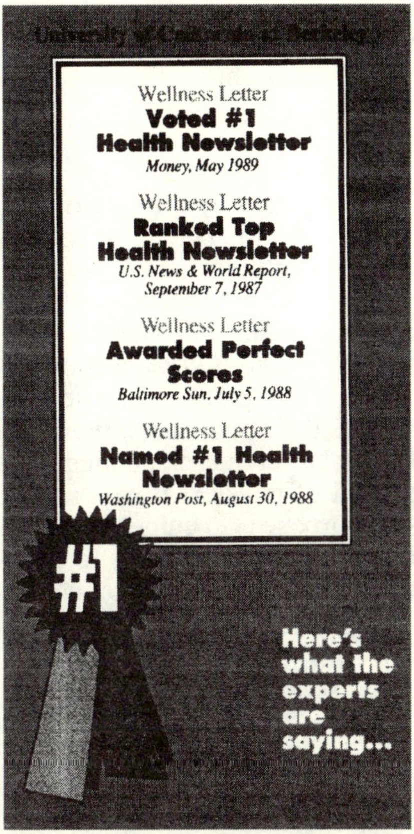

The U.S.News & World Report rating of newsletters was very comprehensive, and, without making a specific reference to any one of the many publications reviewed, I quote a few remarks relative to a few:

"A somewhat elitist magazine....long detailed articles..."
"A poor source of health news...selling health cream..."
"Apparently aimed at young fitness-minded women...headlines

"Apparently aimed at young fitness-minded women...headlines promise more than articles deliver..."

"...pushing vitamins. They also lack depth...scanty clinical articles..."

"An excellent source for the sophisticated consumer."

About the ***University of California Wellness Letter:***

"An interesting, excellent publication that covers a wide variety of health issues...."

(The *Wellness Letter* has also since been voted No. 1 by *Money Magazine* and the *Washington Post,* as well as awarded "perfect scores" by the *Baltimore Sun.*)

I recognize that some who subscribe to other publications, as well as their publishers, will disagree with the above due to the nature or target of each publication and which might also relate to their pursuit of physical fitness and good health. As you will note, my sole purpose is to guide the reader down the path of ***preventive medicine.*** My only advice is to follow your own good judgment along with your doctor's advice in such pursuit.

CHAPTER TWO

MY PATH TO NATURAL NUTRITION

The path to good nutrition was a natural for one who spent his childhood in New England with a mother cooking as her parents and forebears did—wholesome and nutritious foods right off of the farm. Very little processed food and what we have come to refer to as "good home cookin'." ***Preventive medicine*** was just "natural" in those days. The flours were just beginning to be "fortified" by additives because of the removal of the nutritious wheat germ and minerals through processing. It was necessary to lengthen "shelf life" due to lack of refrigeration as we know it now. Today, we are reversing that process but paying expanded fees for health care and exorbitant prices for organic, non-chemical foods in health food stores and super markets. I am not criticizing these prices as a whole for I realize the costs of production in this day and age. However, I do believe that we can find a lower cost supply of the basic foods necessary for good health. Personally, I buy my flour from a local mill and have for years bought grain products from Walnut Acres, Penns Creek, PA, a truly organic farm. The Walnut Acres catalog is almost a textbook of health in itself, and the writings of it's founder, Paul Keene, are always an inspiration. (See Bibliography for address). There are others but you must search them out.

There is no doubt about the high costs of advertising with expensive colored catalogs to be figured into the cost of products we buy. I am familiar with mailing costs of one national organization whose postage sending their monthly magazine has gone from $180,000 in 1970 to nearly $5 million today! When we buy in local stores, prices are controlled by labor, rent and other costs of doing business, so perhaps most of our mail order organizations are justified in their prices. I think that you will know when you are being gouged and can control your costs to a degree. Bear in mind that good health costs money that might have been spent on doctors and other medical expenses.

My mother was right off the farm in Maine, one of four daughters who learned to cook basically nutritious foods grown right on the farm. She fed a working family of five during my childhood—depression years—on a very healthy diet of whole grains, home-grown vegetables, eggs and chicken, as well as "stretching" those left-overs into excellent stews and pot pies. The waters were not polluted then (we lived on the seashore) and our sojourns to the beach resulted in dishes made from clams, oysters and mussels, as well as an abundance of fish—mackerel, flounder, "black" fish (tautog) and hundreds of blue fish, after my older brother got the fishing bug. The chowders, soups and stews were also a part of my gourmet ***preventive medical*** heritage, and, even today there is nothing more tasty than a good stew, fish or clam chowder, made with all those basic vegetables and meat, served with hot fresh bread, rolls or muffins—all easy to make *at very low cost!* A lost art which should be taught in our schools or nutrition classes available to our mass population who have never learned to "stretch a dollar".....similar to the Home Economics classes of earlier education.

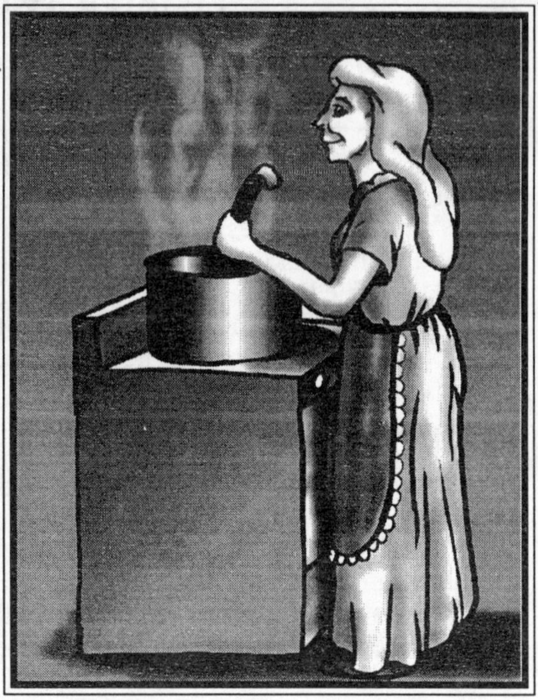

One doesn't need expensive cuts of meat to be healthy. Of course, some of these meals I refer to demand a bit of preparation and work which doesn't appeal to many of the younger generation. This being the age of fast foods, frozen dinners and quick microwaving. I am not averse to commercial preparations of this kind but think that they are easily prepared on your own—and possibly more nutritious—which you can then freeze much cheaper with a great deal more control relative to input from your personal recipes.

Recently, our local paper reported upon a *Newsday* article about a woman in the Home Style Division of the Book Of The Month Club, New York City, who shops and prepares her meals for the week on each weekend. She seems to be doing what we have done for years, even when we had four hungry, active children for whom to prepare meals. I was so interested in her routine that I telephoned to find out if perhaps she might have written a cookbook about her process. She hasn't, but we had a very nice chat about her hobby. Both she and her husband are busy executives, working long hours each day, with little time to prepare healthy, nutritious evening meals upon reaching home. Therefore, she has made doing so into a hobby, cooking and preparing meals in portions for the freezer on the week-end, to be microwaved or reheated conveniently when arriving home.

Think about this if you have never prepared any of your own frozen food dinners or snacks. Buy those containers used for individual or multiple servings and prepare extra when you cook your next main meal, which I'm sure you do once in awhile! Prepare some dishes on weekends, especially if you are working . Then freeze your own at *much lower cost,* using your microwave or oven to thaw and reheat. You will be more than pleased with the results, I assure you, and you have the added advantage of being able to spoon off congealed fat prior to reheating. Remove your planned meal from the freezer to the refrigerator the night before to make life a little easier when returning from a busy day.

There are only two of us to cook for now but we still find ourselves cooking for a larger family so have learned a few tricks such as left-over rice under chili in an individual serving dish, meat balls and spaghetti, chicken dishes and stews all frozen individually. So simple. Dishes too numerous to mention can be prepared this way for future heating in a toaster oven or microwave. Use your imagination!

There are thousands of you "out there" who have no concern about weight or blood pressure in relation to your food intake, but be conscious of the fact that thin people can get high blood pressure and have heart attacks too! Mother Nature or the "Powers That Be" gave us genes which control mentality and health, provided we *listen to what our body is telling us*. It's your obligation to set up your own ***preventive medicine*** practices.

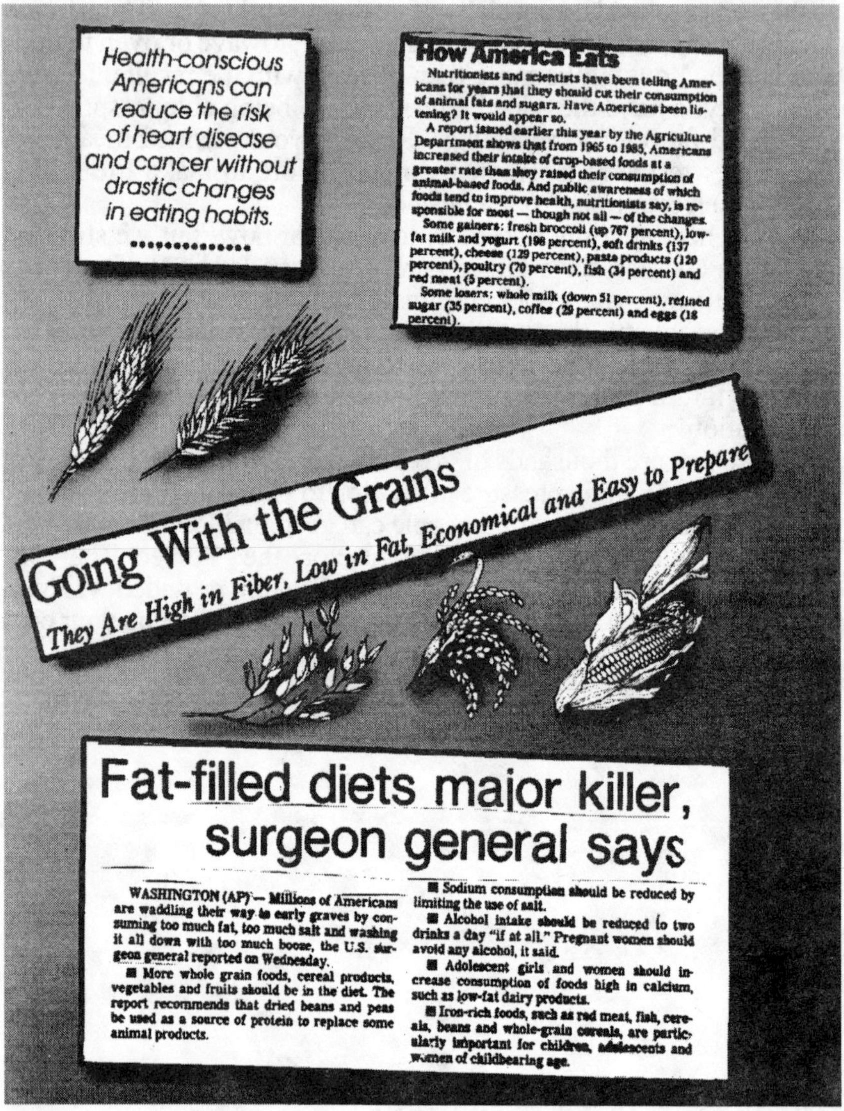

Health-conscious Americans can reduce the risk of heart disease and cancer without drastic changes in eating habits.

How America Eats

Nutritionists and scientists have been telling Americans for years that they should cut their consumption of animal fats and sugars. Have Americans been listening? It would appear so.

A report issued earlier this year by the Agriculture Department shows that from 1965 to 1985, Americans increased their intake of crop-based foods at a greater rate than they raised their consumption of animal-based foods. And public awareness of which foods tend to improve health, nutritionists say, is responsible for most — though not all — of the changes.

Some gainers: fresh broccoli (up 767 percent), low-fat milk and yogurt (198 percent), soft drinks (137 percent), cheese (129 percent), pasta products (120 percent), poultry (70 percent), fish (34 percent) and red meat (5 percent).

Some losers: whole milk (down 51 percent), refined sugar (35 percent), coffee (29 percent) and eggs (18 percent).

Going With the Grains

They Are High in Fiber, Low in Fat, Economical and Easy to Prepare

Fat-filled diets major killer, surgeon general says

WASHINGTON (AP) — Millions of Americans are waddling their way to early graves by consuming too much fat, too much salt and washing it all down with too much booze, the U.S. surgeon general reported on Wednesday.

■ More whole grain foods, cereal products, vegetables and fruits should be in the diet. The report recommends that dried beans and peas be used as a source of protein to replace some animal products.

■ Sodium consumption should be reduced by limiting the use of salt.

■ Alcohol intake should be reduced to two drinks a day "if at all." Pregnant women should avoid any alcohol, it said.

■ Adolescent girls and women should increase consumption of foods high in calcium, such as low-fat dairy products.

■ Iron-rich foods, such as red meat, fish, cereals, beans and whole-grain cereals, are particularly important for children, adolescents and women of childbearing age.

CHAPTER THREE

THE MAGIC OF VITAMIN E

A short publication (booklet) was written and published by J.I. Rodale in 1954, *How To Eat For A Healthy Heart*[8] which, in addition to the Adelle Davis book previously mentioned, changed my life and guided me to a healthy heart through the use of Vitamin E. The outside cover remarks were startling to me, quoting statistics about "Americans dying from heart disease ***five*** times as fast as males in Italy, ***ten*** times as men in Japan!" Since that time great studies have been made in regulating **fat** intake in American diets and I am sure that the relationship between these national statistics has changed. As a matter of fact, I know that it has changed. However, one of the facts recently stated by researchers and published in syndicated newspapers states that the change in diets to more meat and fat in European diets (especially French) will "catch up" with them in the future, possibly resulting in more heart attacks. We'll see. Maybe some new development will come along that wipes out heart conditions completely before that time.

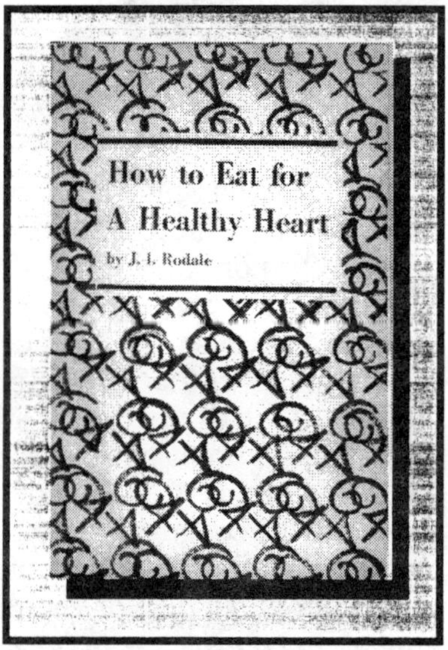

Rodale wrote about the body needs of lecithin, vitamins E, C and calcium as it relates to a healthy heart, and expounded in great detail on Vitamin E as used by the then not-so-famous Doctors Evan & Wilfred Shute in their Canadian clinic. *Time Magazine,* (June 10, **1946**) reported upon the Dr's Shute research, *"heralding" their work on vitamin E as a "new and startling discovery: a treatment for heart disease (the nation's #1 killer), which so far has succeeded against all common forms of the ailment—large concentrated doses of vitamin E—benefited four types of heart ailment (95% of total), arterioschlerotic, hypertensive, rheumatic, old and new coronary heart disease. The vitamin helps a failing heart. It eliminates anginal pain."*

Time, May 31, **1993**, (nearly 50 years later) reported upon the *New England Journal of Medicine* studies involving more than 120,000 people—87,000 female nurses ages 34 to 59, and 40,000 other health other health professionals between ages 40 and 75, over an 8 year period, **all of whom took over 10 times the normal recommended daily allotment (RDA)**. (Researchers are cautious, as is this writer, and do state that no one knows about safety of mega doses of vitamins over the long run, and that there is no substitute for getting plenty of exercise and cutting down on dietary fat).

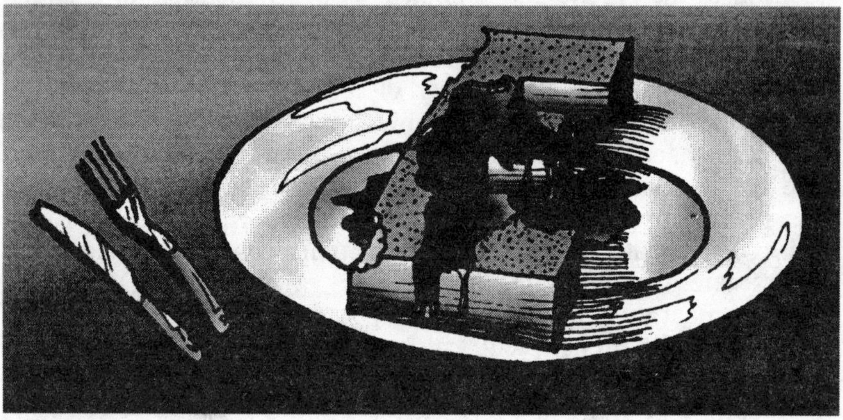

Dr.Evan Shute originally used vitamin E for treatment of habitual abortion successfully. In discovering that vitamin E appeared to delay the normal clotting of blood, he decided to use it on a patient suffering from purpura (bleeding). This patient could not be operated upon because of a heart condition and he found that the addition of vitamin E in the diet helped the heart condition more than the purpura. (One of my doctor advisors, when reading this manuscript was quick to point out that, "biologically, this makes sense for fat-soluble vitamins A, D, E and K are manufactured in the liver and are the key in the coagulation cascade"). That is when the brothers joined forces in treating heart and circulatory patients with their own carefully worked out plan of vitamin E therapy. This was truly the beginning of ***preventive medicine*** as it related to the heart and cardiovascular system.

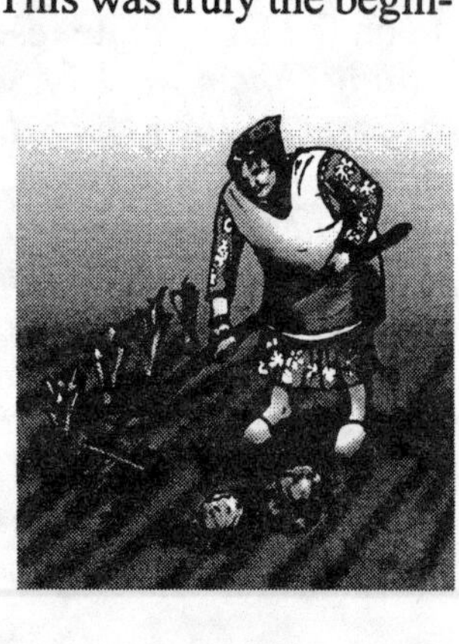

Their next heart patient was their own mother who was so ill that she was unable to walk across the room. According to their own testimony, **she was gardening four weeks after she began to take vitamin E.** A priest was a bed case from phlebitis and was able to resume duties comfortably. A woman who had been in bed for four months with a heart condition, having been told that she would never work again, resumed her job after vitamin E treatment and had been back to her job in a carpet plant for 5 years when Rodale wrote about the doctors successful treatment of patients with the use of vitamin E. But even then the governing body of all physicians and surgeons practicing in Ontario decided *"on evidence submitted, the committee is convinced that vitamin E has no place in the treatment of cardiovascular disease."* Stubborn, weren't they?

The success of their treatment with vitamin E was startling to the degree that when Dr. Wilfred Shute was asked to speak at the Rotary Club in Montreal by a business man member who had been put back on his feet by the Shute treatment, the chairman who was a doctor, flatly refused to invite him to speak. Why? As the Shutes stated, *"evidently the medical opposition was caused by the fact that the doctors considered heart patients as their retirement annuity due to the necessity of continuous treatment."* The Shutes, by that time in the 1950's, had 180 doctors among the 10,000 patients they had treated for heart and circulatory disease! Asked for an explanation of why these doctors were refusing to recognize and prescribe Vitamin E for their patients at that time, the Dr's Shute reply was:

"Some of our loudest critics are taking vitamin E themselves. Many dispense Vitamin E but will not sign a prescription for it. Many doctors returned to their practice on vitamin E after coronaries disabled them but were ashamed to admit the source of their help, even to their closest friends."

Preventive medicine in action by the very people publicly decrying same! (I doubt that the threat of law suits back then, as of today, was the reason.)

At that time, *Macleans,* a Canadian magazine, had assigned a Mr. Eric Hutton to do painstaking research among friends and enemies of vitamin E therapy for heart disease. The resulting figures were amazing. One group of 33 friends who had heart attacks, 20 treated with vitamin E were alive and 13 who had not been so treated were dead.

Among pharmaceutical houses preparing Vitamin E he was told:

* 28% of doctors used vitamin E but would not openly approve of it's therapy.

* Among 800 doctor customers, 228 made enthusiastic comments on the effectiveness of vitamin E in treating heart disease.

* One eminent physicist felt that vitamin E was "the secret armament" of World War II due to increased mental and physical endurance. He refused to speak openly about it because the medical

profession had given the idea that "*anyone who believes in vitamin E is slightly in the screwball class.*"

Of course, things have changed since that time, and this writer has much more confidence in the medical profession than is displayed by these facts and figures. An aside to the Rotary Club refusal was that a subsequent chairman invited Dr. Wilfred Shute to speak. As Rodale wrote, "*The reaction on the part of some medical members of the Rotary was instantaneous. They protested so strongly that the committee finally agreed not to cancel the speech, but to cancel the proposed broadcast of it.*" Later the MD Rotarians tried to prevent the Montreal newspapers from publishing accounts of the speech, but Mr. McConnell, publisher of the *Star*, and members of his staff *who had benefited* from being treated with vitamin E, did so. In addition to defending freedom of the press, the *Star* editorial board was "*defending a friend whose integrity was questioned,*" when they published an editorial about courtesy and controversy, questioning why, "*certain medical men feel so strongly that they are prepared to go to great lengths to prevent public discussion of it" (vitamin E).*

I mentioned previously that my motive in writing this is to pass along benefits from ***preventive medicine*** that I feel have helped me in maintaining a healthy life after a heart attack at age 40. Sometime during the same period of my sales life, there was a pamphlet published by an organization named, *Probe*, in New York City. I was so impressed with the contents that I attached it to the inside cover of my Rodale booklet to act as a continuous reminder of what had already happened to me. The title, *Everyone Can't Have A Heart Attack—But—You Can Try.* A clever title that promoted immediate and continuous rereading which I am sure benefited many salesmen who received copies, for it was certainly true then-and today-to the hazards of the profession of salesmanship. The pamphlet contents:

(The Italics are mine)

* **Fried Chicken & Apple Pie**

Eat thick gravies, French fries, Hollandaise, whipped cream—Help yourself!

* **Forget Your Age**

Work as hard as you did 20 years ago. *(I tried it. It works!)*

* **Run....**

——for trains, buses, airplanes—keep the schedule!
Climb stairs on the double, move furniture, shovel snow.

* **Vacation Telephones**

Telephone the office 2 or 3 times per day. *(You can do it better today with cellular phones—really keep in touch momentarily!)*

* **Spend More....**

——than you make, of course! *(Now we have all those credit cards to help build up worrisome expense!)* Keep yourself "boiling." Constant fretting, anxiety, inadequacy, pillar of the church and community (*though broke!*). You know—do all these things and then.....

You've Made The Club!

Plug away every day, just as a dedicated golfer does! *(You probably belong to a club and have that added expense too).* Suddenly, one day everything works, and, presto! Success, victory, par! You will find yourself a member in good standing of "The Club"—flat on your back in the hospital— *YOU MADE IT!*

As the *Probe* pamphlet finished...Now let's start all over again.

* Whatever your age, be aware of your limitations.
* When you tire, taper off. *(Never exercise when tired).*
* Arrive early for appointments.
* Eat and drink in moderation.
* Have a complete check-up at your doctors at least once a year.

* **The Magic Key**........

The safety slogan of Puerto Rico———

"Reduzca la velocidad y viva mas"——————

SLOW DOWN AND LIVE LONGER !!!

I did just that many years ago, thanks to a smart and compassionate doctor, and am able to pass this advice on to anyone who will listen as I enjoy life and family into my late 70's, as I write this, while practicing what I preach...***Preventive medicine!***

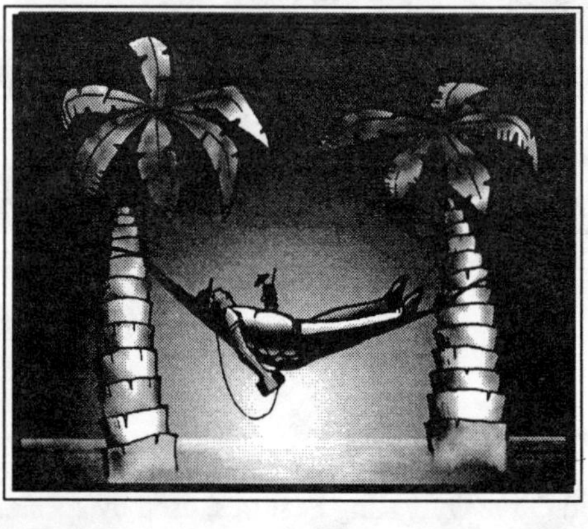

(Note: See Epilogue for latest up-to-date research being done on Vitamin E as reported in *The Wellness Letter.*)

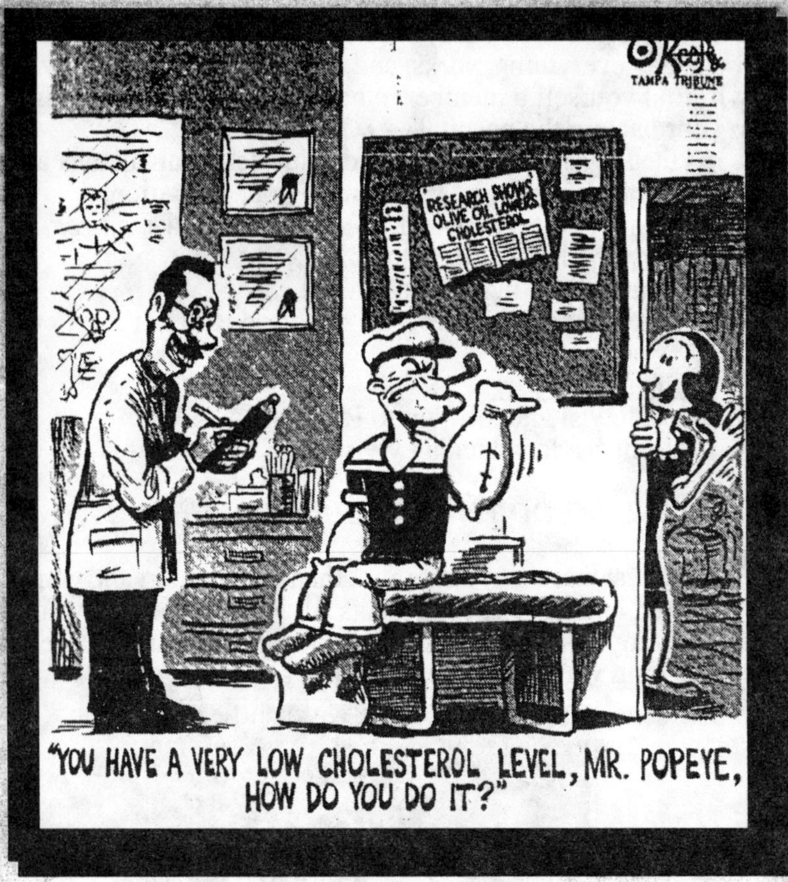
O'Keefe
TAMPA TRIBUNE
RESEARCH SHOWS OLIVE OIL LOWERS CHOLESTEROL
"YOU HAVE A VERY LOW CHOLESTEROL LEVEL, MR. POPEYE, HOW DO YOU DO IT?"

Popeye and Olive Oyl© King Features, used by special permission as it appeared in Tampa Tribune

CHAPTER FOUR

"YOU ARE WHAT YOU EAT"

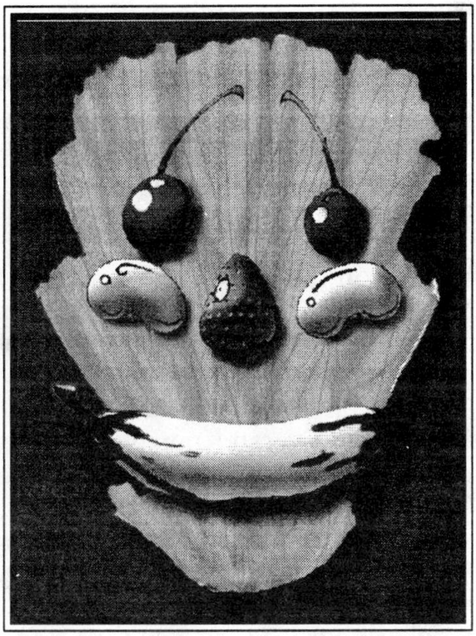

That old plum! I fear that many of us would be sugar plums if this old axiom was completely true. The candy, soda and cereal industry has through the years "educated" us on the "value" of all that sugar in our diets and we are now trying to change it all with low-cal this and light that. I can remember reading some years ago that Hitler was a sugar addict and was considered insane as a result thereof. He did a lot of damage to the world and now we do it to ourselves as we traverse the special supermarket aisle containing all those processed and sugared cereals. A shopper today has to have intelligence enough to skip 99% of these cereals in favor of choosing nutritious, unsugared brands, as well as choose for low sodium content. It's not easy but it can be done with a little perseverance. Of course, if you have the children with you when shopping, that adds another measure of difficulty!

Those processed grains just do not have the nutritional value of plain old oat meal and those other cereals that must be cooked to enjoy. Years ago mother put the oatmeal on the stove the night before, but today you can cook it in the microwave almost as quick as the time it takes to open and pour the processed and less nutritious kind. The instant varieties, however, can contain much higher salt, sugar and fat, as noted by *The Wellness Letter.*[7] I do a batch of regular oatmeal one day and reheat a daily serving portion for one minute in the microwave each morning. I realize that time schedules are important in the morning, but one minute heating same could be arranged if planned that way.

Warning! Cover it so that it doesn't boil over, especially if you add wheatena as I do quite often. Wheatena is an excellent source of *unsalted, unsugared* toasted crushed wheat, bran and wheat germ. What better method of ***preventive medicine*** at breakfast time, that all important first meal of the day to get you and the children off to an excellent nutritious start for the day.

They do sell individual portions that can be cooked in just a minute right in the dish but watch out for that sugar in most of them. Make your own individual portions and save a few dollars. Use skim milk and cut down on the fat intake. I lived through the days of 4% non-homogenized butterfat which was delicious but was probably the beginning of my early clogged arteries with those fatty deposits.

Of course, if you have never learned to use those control buttons on the microwave, and I do hope the reader is not in this category, but, if so, you do have a problem! However, ask an 8-year old for they learn how to use computers and control buttons at an early age in school these days!

I have a great deal of respect for our former U.S. Surgeon General, C. Everett Koop, who was not afraid to "tell it like it is" in respect to most within the confines of his jurisdiction. And he is still doing the same in retirement, having recently spoken out on the subject of many Americans "*waddling*" their way to an early grave.

Now that verbiage is certainly laying it on the line for most of us and should get our attention in a hurry! (I quote from recent article in our local newspaper.) "*Too much fat, too much salt and washing it down with too much booze.*" Diseases of dietary excess and imbalance are among the leading causes of death in the United States. "*Over-consumption is now a major concern for Americans,*" as bluntly stated by Dr. Koop.

Continuing with his advice from the same newspaper article, more whole grain foods, cereal products (and he's not referring to all that sugared stuff), vegetables and fruits, dried beans and peas as a source of protein to replace some of the animal products. Reduce the consumption of fat, especially saturated fats from butter or untrimmed red meat. Alcohol, if at all, should be limited to 2 drinks per day and pregnant women should avoid it completely. Adolescent girls and women should increase consumption of foods high in calcium, such as ***low-fat*** dairy products.

Finally, he issues us all a good warning and bit of advice. Quote:

"*What we eat may affect our risk for several of the leading causes of death for Americans, notably coronary heart disease, stroke, atherosclerosis, diabetes and some types of cancer.* ***These***

disorders together now account for more than two-thirds of all deaths in the United States."

Good nutrition and ***preventive medicine*** begins with those grains previously mentioned, plus fresh or frozen vegetables. So much has been written about broccoli (even though President Bush objected to it), cauliflower, cabbage, kale, brussels sprouts, green onions, that whole family of vegetables rich in anti-cancer **sulphoraphane**, high in fiber, vitamin C and beta carotene, as well as low in fat.

The American Institute for Cancer Research Newsletter[25] reported upon a study of **sulphoraphane** done by Dr. Paul Talalay, MD, who headed the Johns Hopkins University School of Medicine team during 12 years of research on vegetables. The prediction that **sulphoraphane** *will block tumor formation in animals and presumably in man was concluded by this study, partially financed by your contributions to the Institute.* (By contributing, you also can receive their excellent newsletter and a gross of articles pertaining to health. Very worthwhile!) A recent study reported in the *Baltimore Sun*, (early 1994), home of Johns Hopkins University, reinforces these past studies and added to the future hopes of producing some sort of pill containing a synthetic variation of **sulphoraphane** in the laboratory.

What more could one wish for in their diet? And don't forget to mix it with a daily dose of exercise such as a fast walk, a bit of jogging if your so inclined, a game of golf or tennis, hiking, cross country skiing—whatever appeals to you and is enjoyable to you. A walk for health, whether fast or a stroll, to get you out of that chair and away from the TV! Couch potatoes are not healthy vegetables!!

A Cornell University researcher I recently read about recommends a low-fat vegetarian diet as a possible secret to preventing cancer, heart disease, osteoporosis and diabetes. He bases his research on a study made of the dietary habits of 6500 people in 65 counties in China. I'm trying not to be negative or facetious about this bit of research and realize all the work which must have gone into same, but, not all of us are interested in being vegetarians, or, Chinese, for that matter. It has been noted in other studies that our body and gene characteristics are not only different than the Chinese, but other ethnic groups throughout the world. Imagine eating all that rice, day in and day out, just trying to be as healthy as a citizen of that great Communist Empire, deficient in meat and other sources of food which we have learned to enjoy as "common" every day food here in our wonderful Democracy?

If we are going to relate our diets to one ethnic group, let's for a moment think about the Italian diet. It has been noted in a variety of studies, one, some years ago, in the Pocono Mountains of Pennsylvania, heavily populated by Italians, that the pasta-eating and olive oil cooking had produced a much lower rate of heart disease compared to the average American. The reason usually stated is their use of olive oil which is 100% fat of the monounsaturated type containing all that good vitamin E. And it's probably true—but—their life-style for the most part (especially in the past) was very different than ours. Their exercise was working at physically difficult labor and farming and I would assume that the figures will begin to even out now that their life-style has changed considerably.

The younger generation beware, for ***preventive medicine*** does not necessarily allow you to forget that one tablespoon of olive oil, whether virgin or not, contains 12 grams of fat! So how much olive oil may one eat and continue to maintain their recommended weight as suggested by those insurance company weight charts? For cooking and salad dressings, it's great, and I have used gallons of it through the years, but moderation and exercise took care of the excess. Not so, today. No garden to tend, no lawn to mow, no shrubs to trim and no kids to chase, all dictate *moderation!*

I've been pretty general up to this point, so let's get into a specific health measure I have followed for years. I credit a great deal of my health to this, having lost my brother at 38 years of age from a stroke, my sister at 51 under similar circumstances and my father at age 72 from a stroke. If anyone should have lived longer, it should have been both my brother and father. My brother was not one to get much exercise, especially after being named the youngest postmaster in the U.S. at age 21, probably to his detriment from a health standpoint, and my father whose family genes predicted longevity. His father died a few months short of 100, two sisters now 92 and 99, respectively, both with active minds, and a brother who lived into his 90's. But, my dad ate more beef and pork fat than I've ever seen anyone devour, so I guess we'd have to say (sadly) that he committed suicide with a knife and fork.

About now, many of you are asking, "What about his mother?" I didn't mention her for a special reason, but she came from "stock" who lived into the 90's. Mother didn't die a natural death, but was killed at age 58 in our nation's worst airplane disaster up until that time (1947), while taking her first airplane journey to visit her mother in San Francisco who was dying of cancer.

So, let's get on with the specifics of ***preventive medicine*** as it relates to health and *your* potential longevity.

CHAPTER FIVE

"ARTERIAL DISEASE TRACED TO YOUTH"
"AS THE CHILD IS FED, SO GROWS THE EATER."

Headlines such as these in national newspapers "stir my very being" when related to heart and circulatory disease. In these articles researchers are quoted about the early stages of atherosclerosis and hardening of the arteries as being linked to high cholesterol levels in early life.

Apparently, the studies about feeding children a diet overabundant in fat content and excessive calories cause children to form bad dietary habits at a young age, carrying these poor eating habits into adulthood and laying the blame for these bad habits at the doorstep of the parents. I suspect that a great deal can be attributed to this theory when we constantly read about our "average" American being 20% or more overweight. Could it possibly be the parents fault for not having used more dietary caution and not having followed a path related to **preventive medicine**? It's not too late for young parents to initiate a diet of less fat to prevent same happening to those future adults under your care who will face even higher medical costs than we see today.

A newspaper report from the journal *Pediatrics,* was that children still eat too much fat and too little calcium, iron, zinc and vitamin E. (How about that? Vitamin E, one of my favorite subjects!) The report:

82% of the children studied ate more than the recommended

30% of total calories from fat, and that....

30% of children studied fell below the 77% of recommended dietary allowances of these vitamins and minerals of calcium, iron, zinc and vitamin E in their diets.

A study, as reported in another newspaper article, was done by a Dr. William P. Newsman 3rd, and associates, of Louisiana State University, and published in the *New England Journal of Medicine,* in 1986. Interestingly enough, and understandable, was the fact that many experts believed then, and now, that youths who had high cholesterol levels were likely to have "fatty streaks" of cholesterol in their blood vessels. It was felt that the "fatty streaks" are the earliest gross recognizable lesions of atherosclerosis as this report stated.

In the Bogalusa, LA report, the doctors based their research on a study of the cardiovascular health of school children, their cholesterol levels, blood pressure and weights. They also conducted autopsies on 35 youths who had died, mostly from accidents, homicide or suicide, between ages 7 to 24, the average age being 18. All but 6 had "fatty streaks" on the main artery, and those with the most fat buildup had the highest levels of cholesterol.

Five years later, another newspaper report quoted from the *New England Journal of Medicine*....the headline....

"Overweight Teens Have Greater Adult Health Woes"

This later study by the *US Department of Agriculture's Human Nutrition Center* in Boston, was based upon 508 youngsters participating in a Harvard Growth Study of school children in Boston's suburbs, from 1922 through 1935. Participants were interviewed and death records of deceased participants were checked, finding that:

*Men fat as adolescents began to die at a higher-than-average rate by age 45.

*Women overweight as youngsters suffer from a variety of health problems, but, at least into their 70's, appear to live as long as their thinner counterparts as teens.

*Overweight teens as a whole are more likely to encounter problems such as heart disease, colon cancer, arthritis and gout by age 70.

*Overweight teen-age boys and girls were **twice** as likely as thin adolescents to develop heart disease and die by age 70.

*Obese boys were **five** times more likely to develop colon cancer and **twice** as likely to contract gout.

*Overweight girls were **60%** more likely to develop arthritis.

The paper quoted the study director, Dr. Aviva Must:

"There is public message here. It is the importance of pre-

venting lifelong overweight, starting in childhood."

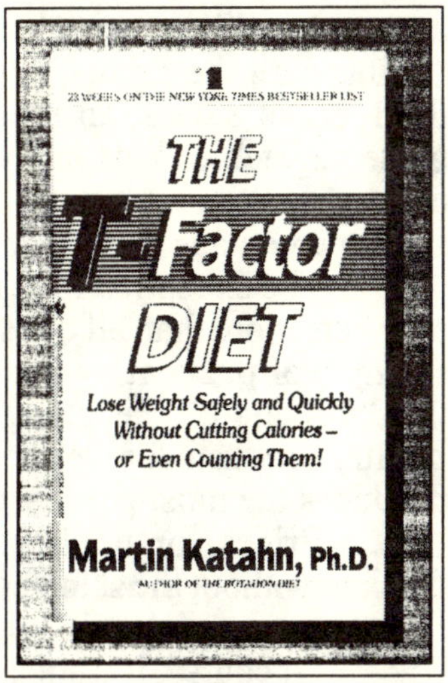

An excellent book, *The T-Factor Diet*[9] by Martin Katahn, PhD, has probably stirred the consciousness of diet-conscious people more than any recent diet book. The "magic" numbers he recommends are a good course of action for any of us to follow for weight loss and is not related to any "fad" diet. His T-Factor formula for weight loss:

* 20 to 40 fat grams per day for women.....

* 30 to 60 fat grams per day for men....

is the best guide I have seen in all my studies of diet and nutrition and is fairly close to the recommended daily fat intake by The American Heart Institute. This guide not only gives you these recommendations, but the book contains excellent fat substitute guides, daily menus, a number of varied recipes to fit anyone's taste, page after page of foods, beverages, salad dressings and desserts in his *Fat and Fiber Content Section.* There is hardly a food or beverage mentioned in his book that one could not use to lose weight if taken in moderation of the fat grams recommended. I call this excellent **preventive medicine!**

Those cereal and fast food ads on TV, aimed at our children and grandchildren, the younger generation, sell these young minds on those high-fat and sugar content foods as good nutrition. Next, as adults, these same individuals are bombarded with ads on TV advising how to lose that 20 extra pounds in just a short period of time, to correct the dietary mistakes of their youth. **But**...The National of Institute of Health concluded, after comprehensive study, that....

90% of those dieters regain the lost weight within 5 years..and that...

Though $30 billion is spent on weight loss programs, Americans have continued to gain over the past 20 years!

The Institute also stated that "weight cycling" or "yo-yo dieting," those bouts of up and down weight gains and losses, could be the cause of other health problems, such as gall stones, heart disease and an increase of uric acid for those afflicted with gout. The better approach, which I am pleased to relate, is followed by my family, "going with the grains," good fresh vegetables daily, especially in the form of salads, an idea my wife and I used as a substitute for those vegetables kids just won't eat (now carried over to the grand-children), skim or low-fat milk, yogurt, cheese, poultry, fish and a small percentage of red meat.

The exception in our family is our 6'7" son-in-law who probably eats more than all our shares of red meat. He does follow a good regimen of **preventive medicine** otherwise, so we have to overlook that "violation." He, along with all the family, does get his share of poultry products for we are fortunate to be living in the county which produces the most poultry of any county in the United States.

Prices for poultry products are reasonable, and cooking chicken without the skin or discarding after cooking does reduce one's fat intake tremendously providing a highly nutritional product.

Of course, it's not as nutritional as truly organic poultry products which are definitely more expensive. However, the feed going to the chicken growers is controlled by the producers of the end product, so we know they are fed a good nutritious diet of whole grains grown right in the area in most cases.

In the past few years, we have seen the estimated cost of cardiovascular disease projected to a tremendous figure. From 1985 to 1986, The American Heart Association estimated that such cost went from **$72 billion** to **$78.6 billion** in just one year. If the increase of **$7 billion** per year was projected to the present (1996), it would indicate that the disease would cost the public an estimated **$142 billion** this year, and continue to escalate throughout our lifetime.

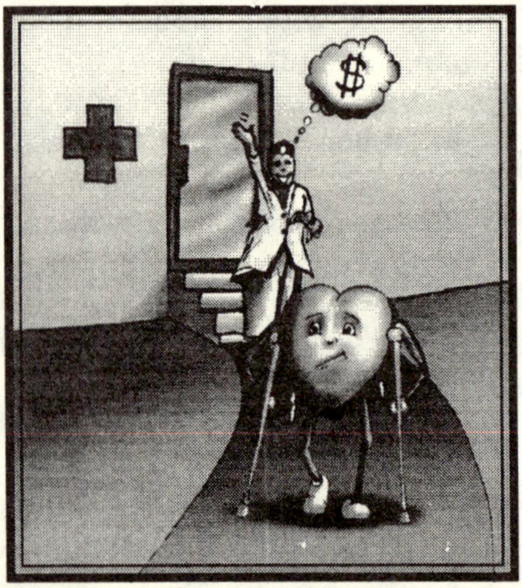

With the high cost of hospitalization, medical procedures and specialization, I can believe the estimates base upon my one day visit to the hospital for minor surgery within the year, approximately $3145 for the hospital, including all those extra charges, doctors' fees and anesthesiologist. One spends more than one day in the hospital when a heart attack strikes! That's why I preach (when I get on my soap box) that a diet containing lecithin and the other basic ingredients recommended by Dr. Rinse, in the following chapters, should be followed as **preventive medicine.**

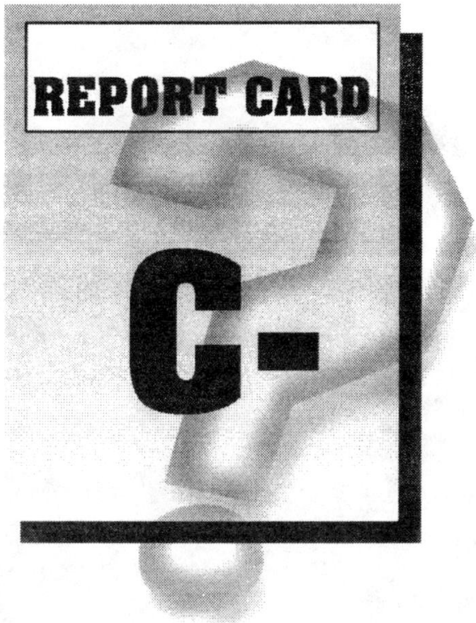

At the time of this writing, there is a proposal in the Maryland legislature to pay for doctors' visits, diagnostic tests and other routine medical care for uninsured children in that state. To quote the Secretary of State:

"The idea is to change the cycle of spending tremendous amounts of money on very expensive care by spending less money up front to keep people from getting sick."

A worthy objective and one which should certainly cut future medical costs. However, it requires a commitment on the part of each individual, as well as any government body.

These reports and statistics relative to our youth of today should make all of us more conscious of the type of food we eat or provide for our children. The most difficult course in life is one of change, to wax philosophical for a moment, whether it be related to diet or any other facet of human endeavor. However, I hope that the following report from the American Health Foundation, a non-profit group, may cause you sufficient concern to make a change in your family diet wherever necessary.

The report gives a sad ***C-Minus*** on the health of our nation's children! In addition to reporting high percentages of mental disorders and attempted suicide, the report states that ***80% of all major illnesses in the United States are related to lifestyle. High-fat diets and physical inactivity are included in a broad range of illnesses and diseases where preventive techniques could raise the grade!***

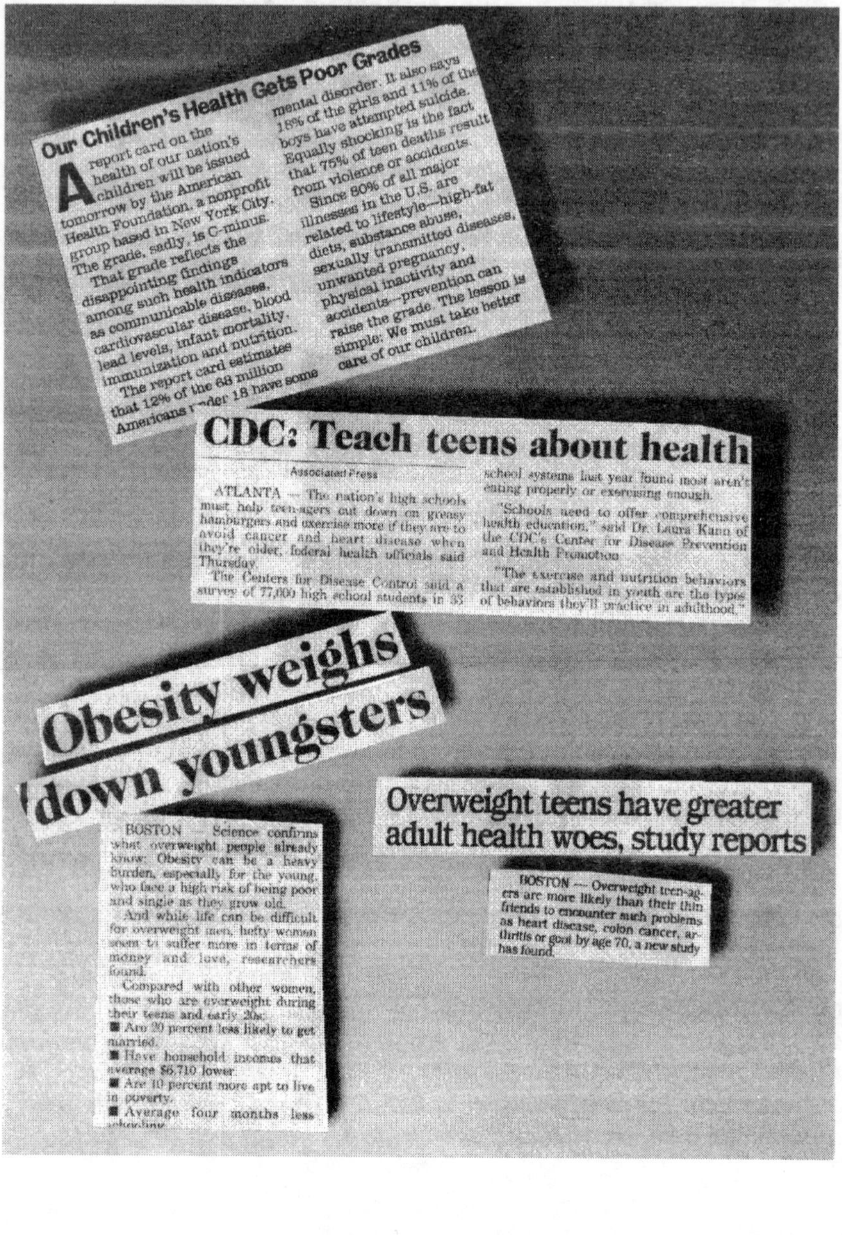

Our Children's Health Gets Poor Grades

A report card on the health of our nation's children will be issued tomorrow by the American Health Foundation, a nonprofit group based in New York City. The grade, sadly, is C-minus.

That grade reflects the disappointing findings among such health indicators as communicable diseases, cardiovascular disease, blood lead levels, infant mortality, immunization and nutrition.

The report card estimates that 12% of the 68 million Americans under 18 have some mental disorder. It also says 18% of the girls and 11% of the boys have attempted suicide. Equally shocking is the fact that 75% of teen deaths result from violence or accidents.

Since 80% of all major illnesses in the U.S. are related to lifestyle—high-fat diets, substance abuse, sexually transmitted diseases, unwanted pregnancy, physical inactivity and accidents—prevention can raise the grade. The lesson is simple: We must take better care of our children.

CDC: Teach teens about health

Associated Press

ATLANTA — The nation's high schools must help teen-agers cut down on greasy hamburgers and exercise more if they are to avoid cancer and heart disease when they're older, federal health officials said Thursday.

The Centers for Disease Control said a survey of 77,000 high school students in 33 school systems last year found most aren't eating properly or exercising enough.

"Schools need to offer comprehensive health education," said Dr. Laura Kann of the CDC's Center for Disease Prevention and Health Promotion.

"The exercise and nutrition behaviors that are established in youth are the types of behaviors they'll practice in adulthood."

Obesity weighs down youngsters

BOSTON — Science confirms what overweight people already know: Obesity can be a heavy burden, especially for the young, who face a high risk of being poor and single as they grow old.

And while life can be difficult for overweight men, hefty women seem to suffer more in terms of money and love, researchers found.

Compared with other women, those who are overweight during their teens and early 20s:

■ Are 20 percent less likely to get married.

■ Have household incomes that average $6,710 lower.

■ Are 10 percent more apt to live in poverty.

■ Average four months less

Overweight teens have greater adult health woes, study reports

BOSTON — Overweight teen-agers are more likely than their thin friends to encounter such problems as heart disease, colon cancer, arthritis or gout by age 70, a new study has found.

CHAPTER SIX

PREVENTION----DR. RINSE

The Rodale book mentioned previously as my introduction to vitamin E as ***preventive medicine*** for cardiovascular conditions, guided my nutritional search for health through the use of foods rich in vitamin E. Corn meal, wheat flour with the wheat germ, safflower and other oils were all used in the muffins and breads baked for the family—and neighbors. (They were unhappy when we left town.) Some years later into my 50's, I began to use the Leahy Clinic in Boston for medical diagnosis and checkups and remember two doctors there commenting on my low cholesterol (at my age). I asked one doctor who had been there 25 years if he had ever heard of the Dr's. Shute and their use of vitamin E in treating for heart and circulatory diseases. No, he had not, so I related my use of corn meal and those other vitamin E foods, while he noted same as I was speaking. I felt quite flattered to have a doctor taking notes as *I* gave the specifics of *my* diet.

I have no recollection of where I obtained my copy of, ***Lecithin,***[4] by Carlson Wade (probably picked it up in a health food store), and was more than *just* interested when reading of Dr. Jacobus Rinse, a world-famous chemist. Dr. Rinse's medical doctor had given him 10 years to live, at age 51, following an attack of angina —but he was jogging daily, at age 81! He had refused to accept the prediction of his doctor, giving him only 10 more years to live, *provided he avoided all physical exertion and continued to take his prescribed medication*, as recommended by his physician.

Dr. Rinse was a chemist and decided to research the disease of the circulatory system to determine *why* he was subjected to these attacks. In his research, Dr. Rinse learned that angina pectoris is comparable to heart failure when the heart does not receive sufficient oxygen. (Now we know why inhaling smoke into our lungs is not a substitute for oxygen!) Angina is caused by fat buildup in the arteries in the form of cholesterol, thereby blocking the circulation of blood. Many years later, cholesterol had become the frightening word in our medical vocabulary!

If fat buildup in the arteries was being caused by diet as suggested in certain studies, then Dr. Rinse surmised that it could also be *changed* by diet—***preventive medicine!*** He reasoned that we feed our cattle and pets a nutritional diet to *prevent* health problems, so why not do the same for the human body? He began to take heavy doses of vitamin C and a multivitamin daily which seemed to be beneficial to his system. About this same time, he learned of the Dr's. Shute of London, Ontario, Canada, and their use of vitamin E in treating patients suffering from heart and circulatory diseases. Through correspondence with them he obtained suggestions that he take 200 milligrams of vitamin E after each meal, which he did for several years, along with the other supplements already being taken, plus garlic. (More on garlic later). As he stated, "*By avoiding strenuous exercise, I managed to live a more or less normal life,*" that is, he did so for the next 5 or 6 years.

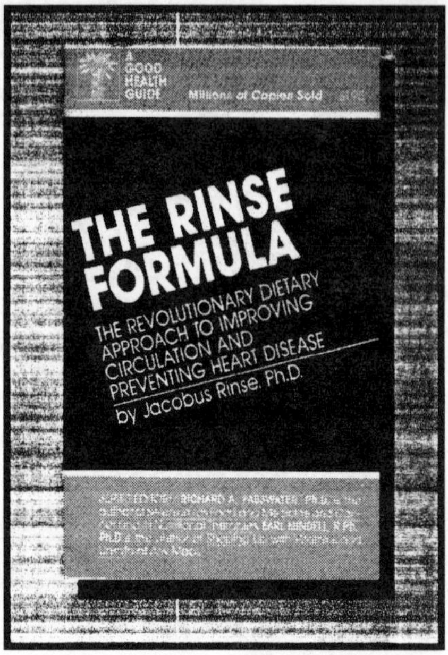

Six years later, however, Dr. Rinse was struck with severe heart pain and frequent recurrence of angina pain. The pain was so bad and recurring so often that he decided to use his knowledge of chemistry and solve this continuing problem through diet. Learning how lecithin had been used in treating animals with heart-cholesterol problems, he began his extensive research on this soy bean derived product and use of same in his diet.

Other researchers were already calling lecithin the "miracle" substance when used with polyunsaturated oils, which were found to liquefy cholesterol deposits in the arteries. Dr. Rinse felt that he was now "onto something," and began his research in earnest while beginning to feel the beneficial results to his own health in only a few days—and—his angina pains had ceased! He also continued with his vitamin C and multivitamin supplements which completely eliminated his angina pains within 3 months! He found that exercising failed to cause any recurrence of same. After months of experimentation and analysis, he devised a breakfast formula including lecithin, wheat germ brewers yeast and a cold pressed linoleate-rich oil as the basis.

What is this miracle formula? Reprinted from the book, ***The Rinse Formula***,[5] by Dr. Jacobus Rinse, copyright © 1981 by Keats Publishing Company, Inc., New Caanan, CT, used with permission:

1 Tablespoon soy lecithin (5 grams)
1 Tablespoon debittered brewer's yeast
1 Tablespoon raw wheat germ
1 Tablespoon dark brown sugar , black strap molasses or raw honey
1/2 Teaspoon bone meal or calcium phosphate (look for lead-free source of bone meal)
or 500 mg calcium oratate or 500 mg magnesium oratate
1 Tablespoon cold-pressed safflower or other linoleate-rich oil, sunflower, corn , or, use sunflower seeds.
Dr. Rinse also takes supplements of these vitamins. The richest source of these vitamins are in parenthesis:
1 gr vitamin C (fresh fruits and vegetables)
50 mg vitamin B6, pyridoxine (fresh salmon, brown rice, banana)
300 mg magnesium oratate or oxide or hydroxide (Brazil nuts, almonds, wheat bran, cashews, lima beans)
50 mg zinc oratate or gluconate or 30 mg zinc oxide (oysters, liver)
200 IU vitamin E(sunflower seeds, wheat germ oil)
50 mcg selenium (yeast)

I have been mixing this so-called "miracle" formula for a healthy breakfast, ***my personal preventive medicine,*** ever since having read about same. I followed the advice of Dr. Rinse, for he states in his book that, *"You can mix it right in your own kitchen."* And you can do it too! I've done it for years and it's no trouble if you do as I do and order all the basics in bulk, the wheat germ, brewer's yeast, lecithin and sunflower seeds (or oil). I am not honestly taking all those other supplements as does Dr. Rinse, but do take some and have a very nutritious diet every day which includes many of those foods mentioned in his personal supplements above.

I use measurements in "parts" of the four basics, lecithin, wheat germ, brewers yeast and ground sunflower seeds, usually measured in cups for a large batch. As a matter of fact, just recently I ground 5 pounds of sunflower seed and then proceeded to mix about

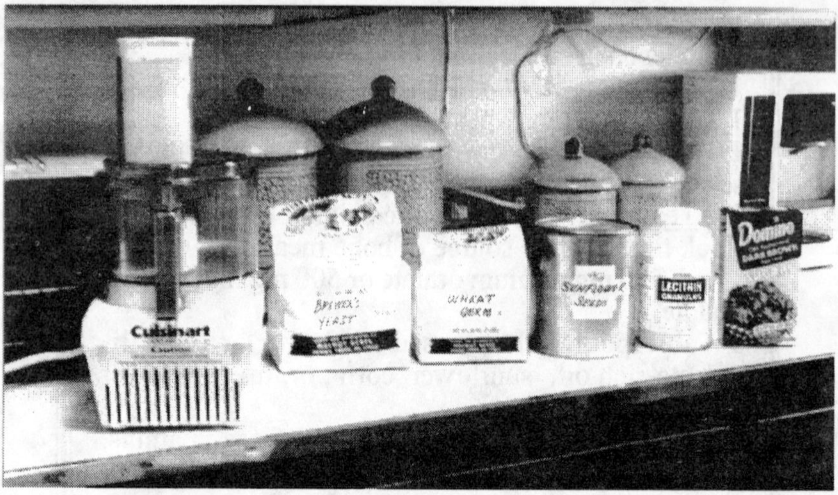

12 pounds of the mix which I will keep refrigerated and use for many weeks to come. A cuisinart or food processor is very handy for this process. I do “donate” it to family members on occasion. I fill a large container for daily use with my oatmeal or other unsugared cereals.

How much should one eat per day? Dr. Rinse’s book shows his original method of 1 tablespoon each of lecithin, brewer’s yeast, wheat germ, brown sugar and linoleate oil or sunflower seeds, and 1/2 tsp bone meal. I use about 1/3 the amount of sugar (you might prefer a sugar substitute) and measure with a coffee scoop—about 2 scoops is equal to one ounce of the mix. You may wish to increase or decrease this amount which you eat on fruit, dry cereal, oatmeal, wheatena--or--even drink it with skim milk. If you make your own bread or muffins, experiment with a half-cup or so in your mix. The hot cereals such as oatmeal and wheatena can be cooked ahead and then individual portions may be reheated daily in your microwave.

There is a company manufacturing the mix, but I find their price very high for a small 14-ounce can, which they advertise “sufficient for two weeks.” Not so if you use it as we do in our baked mixes, pan cakes, muffins, breads, as well as in our hot and cold cereals. I find that I can buy at catalog prices, from establishments such as Walnut Acres, the basic lecithin, wheat germ, brewer’s yeast and sunflower seeds, and that I can mix 2 pounds for approximately $7.00. That is less than one-quarter the price of the advertised mix which does have added some of the supplements Dr. Rinse takes daily. With your own basic mix, take one or two good vitamin tablets per day—or even better—eat some of those foods he mentions, if you are not already doing so—bananas, brown rice, nuts, etc., in amounts depending on your necessary caloric intake, and, following this ***preventive medicine*** agenda, you shouldn't need too many extra pill supplements.

There is a sweetener on the market which might interest you as one searching for organic foods, Sucanat, cold-pressed organic sugar. Invented by an eminent European pediatrician, who did so when noting his children patients were having what he considered too much tooth decay from processed sugar. This, in place of brown sugar, is highly nutritious but more expensive. Molasses or honey are great substitutes and I use very little sweetener as a general rule. Of course, diabetics can have very little, if any, of these sweeteners. When mentioning these liquid sweeteners, honey or molasses, they are, of course, used separately. Don't try to mix them with the dry ingredients in bulk or you are going to have a real mess!

Raw wheat germ seems to give an "uncooked" flavor to me, so, after reading in the *Handbook of Nutritional Contents of Foods,* prepared by researchers for the United States Department of Agriculture, that the cooking process in baking caused less than 20% loss in some minerals, a 60% gain in vitamin A, a 27% loss in sodium and a 44% gain in potassium, I decided that toasted wheat germ was more palatable to my taste and just as beneficial. *The same publication indicated that toasting a piece of cracked wheat bread increased every measure of vitamin/mineral content available for digestion.* (Said publication now replaced with more comprehensive books covering the nutritional value of foods and available for purchase from the U.S. Department of Agriculture, Washington, DC.)

The use of sunflower seeds in place of oil, which is not the most pleasant "oily" taste for breakfast (why suffer?), gives you all the oil content needed to work with the lecithin to provide the beneficial effects desired, for sunflower seeds contain 50% oil and have a pleasant "nutty" flavor. I cannot find a supply of ground sunflower seeds so I buy 5 pounds at a time and grind them all at once (as previously mentioned). A bit tiresome but it's done, once and for all, and the supply lasts many weeks. A little time and effort devoted to ***preventive medicine.*** By the way, I keep all these grains either refrigerated or in the freezer for preservation.

There has been no explanation of "cold-pressed" oils for those of you never having encountered the words in relation to purchasing vegetable oil. Most oils sold in the market place are produced by a **heat process** to release the oil from it's natural environment. The *cold-pressed* process uses no heat but the product is pressed cold to obtain the oil in it's natural state. The heat used in processing oil is known to reduce the vitamin E content of the end product, therefore, when purchasing oil, look for oil produced by a cold-pressed process. It's more expensive but you need to use less for the same results.

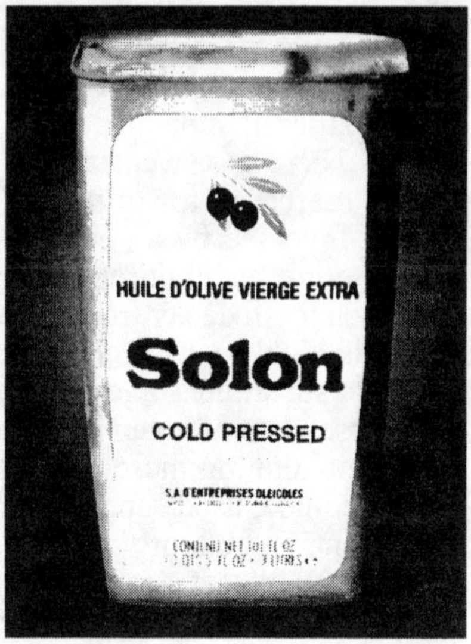

One day, while mixing the basics, I decided that I would like to meet Dr. Rinse, if he was still alive. It took a few letters and follow-ups but I finally met with him at his home in East Dorset, VT, when he was 86 years of age. He was alive, alright! My wife and I enjoyed a wonderful visit and lunch with Doctor and Mrs. Rinse, as well as a few hours of healthful conversation. We walked through the woods trying to keep up with his fast pace, passing the pond where he and Mrs. Rinse had been swimming that same morning—early October in Vermont!

During our conversation I asked, "Do you still jog daily?" His reply, *"No, but I take fast walks and RUN some of the time while going to the Post Office* (nearly 2 miles away). *I really don't need that kind of exercise with my wood chopping and all the other work I do around these 65 acres."* I can attest to the veracity of his statement, for I was shown his 3-year supply of logs he was cutting and splitting daily.

We visited with Dr. Rinse again in the summer of 1992 and had a wonderful afternoon visit, discussing various topics related to health as we sat outside his home amid the beautiful mountains of Vermont. It was after this visit that he reviewed my writings in great detail, writing me a full page of ideas to encompass within these pages. We were deeply saddened by his sudden death about one year later, at age 93. However, his research and formula will live on forever.

I have endeavored to outline the basics of this ***preventive medicine*** formula herein. However, I think that anyone having had their interest "sparked" relative to reducing their chance of heart or circulatory disease should acquire a copy of the book, ***The Rinse Formula***[5] by Jacobus Rinse, PhD. You will learn more about the study of atherosclerosis, and the consequences of vitamin and mineral deficiencies, as outlined by this world-famous chemist. And you get all this for only $1.95—probably at your health food store. What a bargain! And it took a heart attack to awaken me to all of this!

To believe that the use of these basic ingredients of lecithin, brewer's yeast, wheat germ and sunflower seed (oil) is a cure-all is an injustice to one's intelligence, but used as a basis for one's basic nutritional body needs is not a bad "foundation" from which to start one's search for health and longevity! The charts presented later in the book certainly show that many of the vitamins and minerals required for your body's well being and health are contained in these basic ingredients.

In a 1988 *U. S. News & World Report*, a noted cardiologist, speaking on the subject of "Cholesterol" before a convention of his peers stated:

"The first thing I ask my patients is...........

WHAT DO YOU EAT FOR BREAKFAST?"

How do ***you*** start ***your*** day?

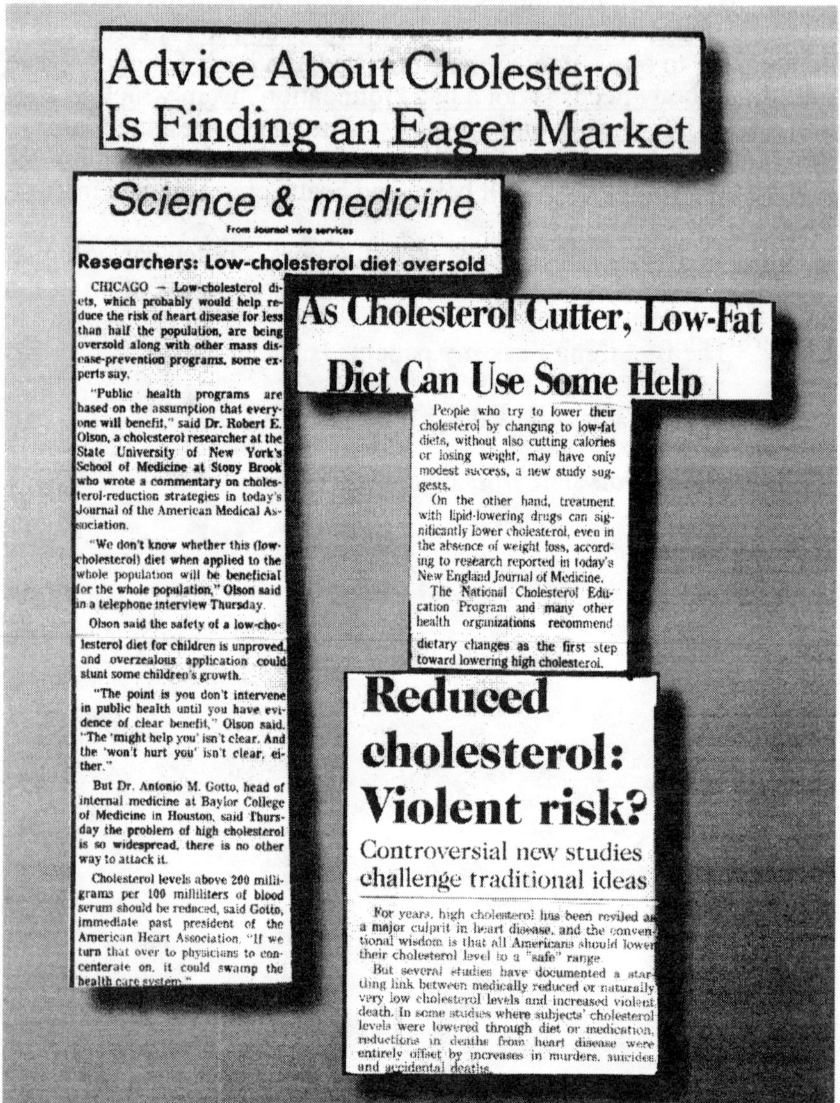

Advice About Cholesterol Is Finding an Eager Market

Science & medicine

From Journal wire services

Researchers: Low-cholesterol diet oversold

CHICAGO — Low-cholesterol diets, which probably would help reduce the risk of heart disease for less than half the population, are being oversold along with other mass disease-prevention programs, some experts say.

"Public health programs are based on the assumption that everyone will benefit," said Dr. Robert E. Olson, a cholesterol researcher at the State University of New York's School of Medicine at Stony Brook who wrote a commentary on cholesterol-reduction strategies in today's Journal of the American Medical Association.

"We don't know whether this (low-cholesterol) diet when applied to the whole population will be beneficial for the whole population," Olson said in a telephone interview Thursday.

Olson said the safety of a low-cholesterol diet for children is unproved, and overzealous application could stunt some children's growth.

"The point is you don't intervene in public health until you have evidence of clear benefit," Olson said. "The 'might help you' isn't clear. And the 'won't hurt you' isn't clear, either."

But Dr. Antonio M. Gotto, head of internal medicine at Baylor College of Medicine in Houston, said Thursday the problem of high cholesterol is so widespread, there is no other way to attack it.

Cholesterol levels above 200 milligrams per 100 milliliters of blood serum should be reduced, said Gotto, immediate past president of the American Heart Association. "If we turn that over to physicians to concenterate on, it could swamp the health care system."

As Cholesterol Cutter, Low-Fat Diet Can Use Some Help

People who try to lower their cholesterol by changing to low-fat diets, without also cutting calories or losing weight, may have only modest success, a new study suggests.

On the other hand, treatment with lipid-lowering drugs can significantly lower cholesterol, even in the absence of weight loss, according to research reported in today's New England Journal of Medicine.

The National Cholesterol Education Program and many other health organizations recommend dietary changes as the first step toward lowering high cholesterol.

Reduced cholesterol: Violent risk?

Controversial new studies challenge traditional ideas

For years, high cholesterol has been reviled as a major culprit in heart disease, and the conventional wisdom is that all Americans should lower their cholesterol level to a "safe" range.

But several studies have documented a startling link between medically reduced or naturally very low cholesterol levels and increased violent death. In some studies where subjects' cholesterol levels were lowered through diet or medication, reductions in deaths from heart disease were entirely offset by increases in murders, suicides and accidental deaths.

CHAPTER SEVEN

CHOLESTEROL & YOU

Following the afore-mentioned research by Dr. Rinse, he wrote a treatise in 1986, *The Absorption of Cholesterol*,[24] which he sent me with verbal permission to use in my writings. I would love to include the whole technical work, and that is the only reason I am not doing so—*technical.* He documented his work by references to studies made by many experts in the fields of medicine and science. A brief and condensed outline- the question:

Is it desirable to lower the cholesterol content of the blood?

* Excessive lowering of cholesterol has increased chances of cancer in many cases.

* Cholesterol has been found by many researchers not to be the **cause** but the **consequence** of deficiencies of lecithin, linoleate oils, vitamins and minerals in the diet.

* Cholesterol is only absorbed in the intestinal wall if the accompanying amount of lecithin is small.

* The duo cholesterol-lecithin is transported in the blood by lipoproteins, now known by their densities as HDL and LDL (high and low density) lipoproteins. A high amount of HDL is a favorable factor while high LDL indicates the possibility of atherosclerosis. The controlling factor is the amount of phospholipids (lecithin) in relation to the cholesterol.

* The variation of lipids with age has been investigated by D. Adlersberg with 1100 men in ages from babies to old age. He found high lecithin in the babies and a gradual decrease with advancing age. On the other hand, with cholesterol, a gradual increase with advancing age was observed.

* Prior to Dr. Rinse's experiments and self-treatment in 1957, patients being prescribed lecithin had not been advised to use a linoleate oil, which is now being done throughout the world.

* It is recommended that older persons add lecithin, linoleate oil, vitamins and minerals to their diets for inhibiting cholesterol absorption and improvement of brain functions. Avoiding cholesterol-containing foodstuffs is not necessary and can even be detrimental to one's health.

All references to the Dr. Rinse treatise are listed in the bibliography.

Studies as reported in the *Readers Digest* 5 or 6 years ago on lipoproteins were most comprehensive, and, admittedly, "more

HOW ATHEROSCLEROSIS AFFECTS THE ARTERIES

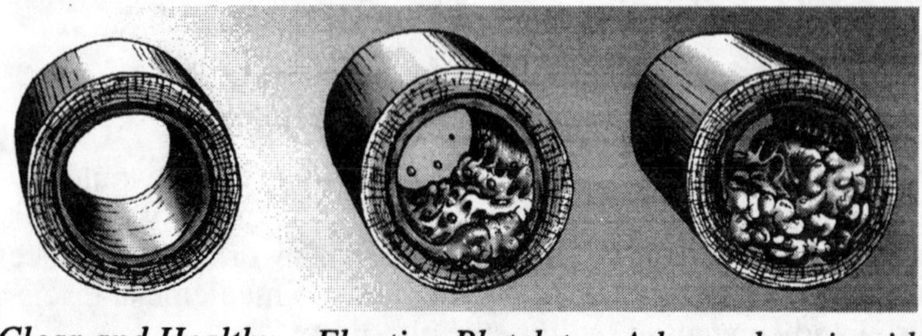

Clear and Healthy Artery | *Floating Platelets and Platelets* | *Atherosclerosis with Plaque Buildup*

investigation is necessary." However, the raising of high density lipoproteins (HDL), the "good" cholesterol over the low density (LDL) is definitely a good procedure to follow, whether it is accomplished through medication prescribed by a physician or by diet as mentioned herein.

* Men between ages 25 to 55 should endeavor to keep their cholesterol level below 240 for less risk of a heart attack. Older men from 160 to 200, if no other health or risk factors are present.

* Women, pre-menopausal, with levels of 240 and above, have less risk of coronary heart disease than men with the same level. Post-menopausal women with high cholesterol levels have approximately the same risk as men, but at older ages the risk decreases. Since that time, a study reported in the *New England Journal of Medicine* supporting the studies and writings of numerous doctors and nutritionists throughout the United States also came to the **same conclusion as Dr. Rinse:**

* Cholesterol risks are overstated except for smokers and those with excessively high blood pressure.

* Possible increase in cancer and strokes as an adverse consequence of low cholesterol.

* Difficult to lower cholesterol by diet.

* Drugs used to lower cholesterol can have unanticipated side effects.

In February, 1993, *The New York Times* reported upon a study published in the *Journal of the American Medical Association* about cholesterol testing. Dr. Stephen P. Hulley and his colleagues at the University of California at San Francisco wrote that there is no justification for routine cholesterol testing in men before age 35, and in women prior to age 45. This study stated their reasoning that endeavoring to reduce cholesterol by use of drug dependency might outweigh the benefits in low-risk people.

Criticism of this study by other medical researchers was "misguided" stated Dr. C. David Naylor, of the University of Toronto, in his editorial accompanying Dr. Hulley's article. Quoting Dr. Naylor in the New York Times article:

"There is a narrow window where cholesterol testing and treatment makes sense—in the middle-aged until around age 70."

The author's interpretation of this controversial study is that you may have your cholesterol tested at earlier ages than suggested by this study, but be cautious of any prescribed drugs to lower your cholesterol at an early age. Change your dietary habits and you might possibly accomplish the same result in a much more healthy manner!

So much for cholesterol, and to quote Dr. Rinse, *"Let's put the cholesterol worry to sleep."* Provided, of course, you are not in the high-risk category, and that you keep those high-density lipoproteins (HDL) fighting to reduce the (LDL) ones in your blood stream.

We can put the worry to sleep but that doesn't preclude all the studies continuously being done in Britain, as well as the United States, as now being reported (See Epilogue).

In late studies now being reported in the *American Heart Association Journal* and *British Medical Journal*, studies covering thousands of people, they give us more worry about very low cholesterol levels, including higher incidence of suicides among tested groups with very low cholesterol. Also, that cholesterol levels below 160 mg per deciliter were associated with stroke, liver and pancreatic cancer, cirrhosis of the liver, as well as—alcoholism! It would seem that from all of these studies a level of from 160 to 240 would possibly keep us healthy—that— and having grandparents with good genetics!

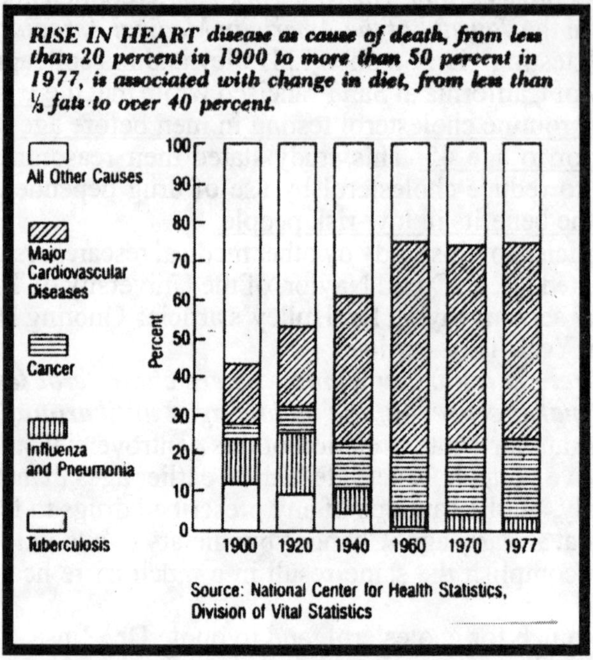

***RISE IN HEART** disease as cause of death, from less than 20 percent in 1900 to more than 50 percent in 1977, is associated with change in diet, from less than ⅓ fats to over 40 percent.*

THE PREVIOUS CHAPTERS PROVIDED THE READER INFORMATION ON WHOLE GRAINS AND VITAMIN E IN THE FOODS MENTIONED. YOU NOW COME TO WHAT SCIENTIFIC RESEARCHERS REGARD AS "THE MAGIC INGREDIENT" IN THESE FOODS SO THE AUTHOR SUGGESTS THAT YOU DO NOT "BREEZE THROUGH" THE NEXT CHAPTER.

LECITHIN IS A NATURAL INGREDIENT THAT IS BEING ACTIVELY RESEARCHED FOR ITS RELATIONSHIP TO GOOD HEALTH. TODAY'S HEALTH-CONSCIOUS CONSUMERS SEEK OUT PROCESSED FOODS THAT ARE MADE WITH LECITHIN INSTEAD OF THOSE MADE WITH CHEMICAL ADDITIVES. IT IS A RICH SOURCE OF POLYUNSATURATED FATS AND IS CHOLESTEROL-FREE.

CHAPTER EIGHT

LECITHIN

One prominent health writer wrote that most in the category of health writers feel that medical science is often finding studies that have previously shown the nutritional value of certain foods. They are "re-discovering," so to speak, medical knowledge previously attributed to the nutritional value of **lecithin**, to use one food as an example. In writing about **lecithin,** this was emphasized by quoting from studies reported upon from 1948 to 1977, and other years prior to the "sudden discovery" of the nutritional value of **lecithin** by certain researchers and prominent writers of later years.

In reading one report, I was more than pleased to note the inclusion of a reference to lecithin in the 1965 Adelle Davis book, *Let's Get Well,*[10] which was one of the first books on ***preventive medicine*** to be placed in my so-called library. Studies reported in leading medical and scientific publications by doctors and researchers worldwide, have been used to prove the value of lecithin in many areas of medicine—and psychiatry.

These studies by doctors in Germany reported, back in 1979, that alcoholic fatty liver has been helped by the phosphatidyl choline in lecithin where cirrhosis has been found in the liver, even in patients with cirrhosis who do not drink alcoholic beverages. One doctor had great results in treating blood clotting problems in patients, one in particular, who had been a "bleeder" for over 20 years. This patient had normal bleeding time in just a few weeks of his prescribing in the diet—phosphatidyl choline from lecithin.

A prominent psychiatrist in New York reported impressive results using lecithin in treatment of patients who were starting to lose memory or having difficulty in remembering names of friends. We recognize this as the beginning of senility in older age, I believe. Just think of that—a nutritional approach to psychiatry!

What is lecithin? Previous chapters outline the dietary use of lecithin and it's seemingly miraculous benefits. Lecithin is a naturally occurring group of phospholipids that is found in nearly every living cell. Though the word lecithin is derived from the Greek, lekithos, which means "yolk of an egg," the primary source of lecithin comes from the soybean.

Writing about the yolk of the egg as being source of cholesterol which has frightened the populace into believing that those of us who continue to eat eggs are loading our arteries with undiluted plaque. This might be the place to advise of a 1954 study mentioned in the Adelle Davis book where patients in the Almeda County Hospital were given fat from egg yolks equivalent to 36 eggs daily, and in no case did the blood cholesterol rise above normal. The yolk fat supplied lecithin and the B vitamin choline which Mother Nature put into the egg and was believed to have the offsetting effect on the cholesterol. For the general population which has been warned to reduce the use of eggs in the diet, this may not sound acceptable, but the results of the study can not be discounted completely. There is no doubt about the high number of fat grams therein, so perhaps the reduction is necessary for those of us who are weight conscious.

Lecithin is used in the food industry as a multi-purpose tool, an emulsifier and "wetting agent" which controls product viscosity. It is a natural ingredient used in processed foods *in place of chemical additives*, and is the reason that we search out processed foods that contain this ***natural*** ingredient. Doctors and researchers hesitate to call it a "miracle food," but results they have attained certainly prove beyond a doubt the true nutritional value of lecithin.

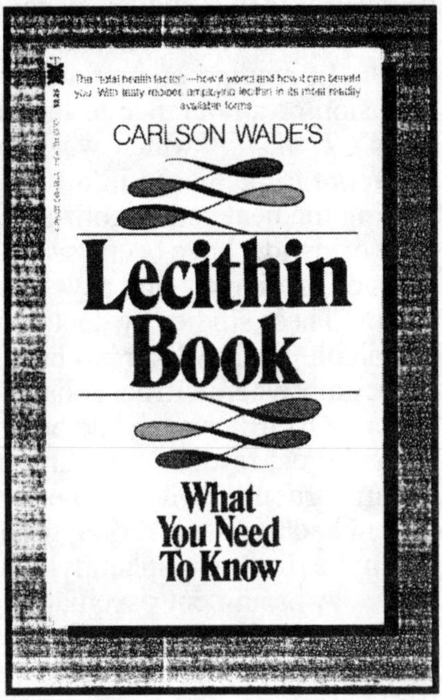

I might add, from my observation of the results of some of these studies, that it would be wise for all of us to plan the inclusion of lecithin in our daily diets, and the younger we begin, the better! Start early in life! Don't wait until you have neurological problems, have a heart attack, angina, high blood pressure or become senile. Of course, that TV add told you, *"If you become senile, don't worry about it because you won't know it!"* Humorous, when stated that way, but not so funny to the family which has to meet the financial obligation of this illness, to the tune of $30,000 to $40,000 per year in a nursing home.

In all of this research on lecithin, PC (phosphatidyl choline), was the important ingredient. Soybeans, being the dominant source of lecithin, are a major crop and source of income to farmers throughout the United States, though I understand from recent reports that our market is being jeopardized by Brazilian and other country imports.

Soybeans are 39% oil and 61% phospholipids, with phosphatidyl choline having the most beneficial effect, so the higher the percentage of PC, the more beneficial the lecithin. The importance of using the granules as a food supplement, as previously mentioned, is that one tablespoon of granules equals the dietary value of TEN of the oil capsuls. In addition, the capsuls usually contain approximately 39% soybean oil which could, in such large amounts, act as a laxative.

Though I did not mention the nutritional value of brewer's yeast in a previous chapter, the same comparison could be made relative to the number of vitamin B tablets one would have to devour to equal one tablespoon of brewer's yeast—the one food containing nearly every vitamin B element. By eating sufficient pills and capsuls to accomplish the same level of the tablespoons of both lecithin and brewer's yeast, one could become quite busy just earning sufficient capital to pay for same. As *The Wellness Letter* states about Vitamin E in the Epilogue, the ones receiving the most benefit would be the manufacturers!

Based upon the current direction of lecithin research, the focus seems to point towards the prophylactic role in potential minimization of high cholesterol reduction and age-related memory problems. Perhaps this summary of it's role in human nutrition will be the catalyst which moves the reader to concentrate on including lecithin into one's daily diet. In so doing, it could become the "beginning primer" to follow in your pursuit of health and longevity—a long and healthy life defying the actuarial tables—and perhaps overriding your expected longevity from your genetic makeup.

As was stated by a noted dietician:

"WE DIDN'T GET TO CHOOSE OUR PARENTS, BUT WE CAN DO SOMETHING ABOUT OUR DIET."

THE FOLLOWING CHAPTER IS SHORT BUT FULL OF NUTRITION. BEANS ARE, OF COURSE, IN THE FAMILY OF LEGUMES, AN ENORMOUS GROUP OF PLANTS IN WHICH THE SEED DEVELOPS IN THE PODS THAT SPLIT OPEN WHEN MATURE. ALL EXCEPT THE THE LONELY SNOW PEA ARE SHELLED FOR HUMAN CONSUMPTION. MOST ALL THE DRY BEANS CAN BE REHYDRATED BY SOAKING AND USED IN "A THOUSAND RECIPES," INCLUDING FAMOUS NEW ENGLAND BAKED BEANS WHICH THIS AUTHOR ENJOYED EVERY SATURDAY NIGHT, WITH LEFTOVERS SERVED AT SUNDAY MORNING BREAKFAST WITH HOT BISCUITS, ETC. IF YOU ARE NOT A USER OF LEGUMES IN YOUR COOKING, THINK ABOUT ENCOMPASSING SOME FORM IN YOUR FUTURE DIET FOR GOOD ECONOMICAL NUTRITION.

CHAPTER NINE

BEANS and LEGUMES

We have discussed grains and vegetables which reduce cholesterol and possibly lower the risk of cancer. Let us not overlook the major source of lecithin, **soybeans,** and the many other **beans** *and* **legumes** which are not only a great source of vitamins and minerals in our diets, but, also a low-cost budget item very high in nutritional value and an excellent substitute for meat.

An excellent article in *American Health, March* 1986,[26] by Gail Levy, M.S.,R.D., nutrition writer and dietitian, covered these "nutritional wonders" (her expression) at great length, outlining their values in supplying Iron, Zinc, Potassium, and vitamin B-6 in diets; the need for less insulin to control blood sugar due to digestive slowness, which causes gentle rises in blood sugar compared to other carbohydrates such as bread and potatoes; the lowering of blood cholesterol due to the lack of total fats, saturated fats and cholesterol; the legume fiber's special quality that forms a gel that binds with cholesterol, which then passes harmlessly out of the body, and the containment of "protease inhibitors" that interfere with protein-digesting enzymes.

In her article, Gail Levy mentioned how "protease inhibitors" were used successfully at the Howard School of Public Health on laboratory animals in preventing tumorous cancers from appearing on their cheeks, after having given the hamsters a chemical which causes oral cancer.

Back about the same time, *Readers Digest* published an excellent article entitled, *The Bean of a Thousand Guises,* by Jack Denton Scott, extolling the many virtues and uses of soybeans, soybean oil (cold-pressed, of course!) tracing the origin back about 3000 years in China. Today, thanks to our specialists work and their collections of plants and seeds, there are over 7000 strains at the University of Illinois Agricultural School.

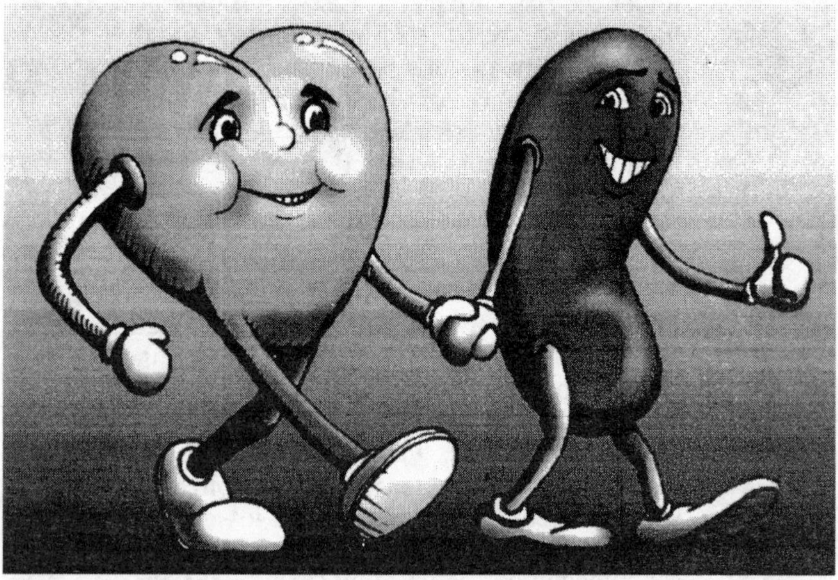

I only remember, when very young, of reading about Henry Ford having made his steering wheels from soybean fiber, but his research was much more comprehensive as noted in the above-named article. Henry Ford even wore a soybean suit, shirt, tie and hat! Soybean fiberboard was in his plans to make a "vegetable car" until a goat ate the license plate made of the fiberboard! A good story and worth repeating!

In foods, tofu, cheesecake, meat loaf, soy burgers and many other uses of soybeans as a substitute for meat have been utilized. You may be familiar with these foods if you frequent health food stores as I have done for the past 30 or more years.

All of these beans and legumes—Pinto, Navy, Kidney, Great Northern, Black Turtle, Black-eyed Peas, Split Peas and Lentils—can be found in your super market at reasonable cost, and their use in your ***preventive medicine*** diet as a meat substitute, as recommended by Dr. Koop, can be most beneficial to your health as well as reducing your budgetary outlay for groceries. Two or three varieties are excellent in soups and stews, especially ministrone soup which can be a meal by itself, full of fresh vegetables and a good beef and/or chicken broth base.

Beans have a reputation for being hard to digest (flatulence in many cases), but, if soaked properly overnight in the refrigerator or three hours at room temperature, then discarding the soaking water to eliminate the raffinose sugars, one can gradually adapt the unaccustomed digestive system to handle this high-fiber food. I even use canned beans when time is of essence, but am careful to eliminate the greater amount of sodium by rinsing in a colander.

Before closing on this mostly nutritious family to include in your everyday diet, I know there are many cook books and magazines on the market containing recipes using beans, or already in your "kitchen library," but I strongly recommend (if you can find it) a book entitled, *Beans & Peas,* 1981.[27] This is a complete guide to their use, including many, many great bean and pea recipes. (There is also an up-to-date cook book on beans, by Choate 1992, mentioned in the Bibliography.)

You can bake them (get a good New England baked bean recipe with nutritious black strap molasses), boil and stew them to make your favorite bean dip with garlic and spices, jalapeno peppers and chili powder, as my son did while in New Mexico. Add cumin, provolone cheese, sour cream (light, of course!). Just use your imagination! Using a chicken or beef broth base, or a ham hock or two, make delicious bean soup with celery, tomato, onions, garlic, carrots, peppers and any other vegetable you might want to add. Don't forget the vegetables with the **sulphoraphane**—cabbage, brussel sprouts, broccoli, kale, green onions, the whole family!

"BEAN" APPETITE!

GARLIC
A NEW PERSPECTIVE

Treasured since prehistoric times, garlic is quite versatile. It is rich in odorous sulfur compunds and has been used in treating a broad spectrum of medical conditions. For modern man, garlic may have more critical contributions i.e., protection from cardiovascualr diseases, toxic pollution, radiation and oxidation. Have you ever wished for a unique food that can help maintain optimum health? Garlic is perhaps one of these foods.

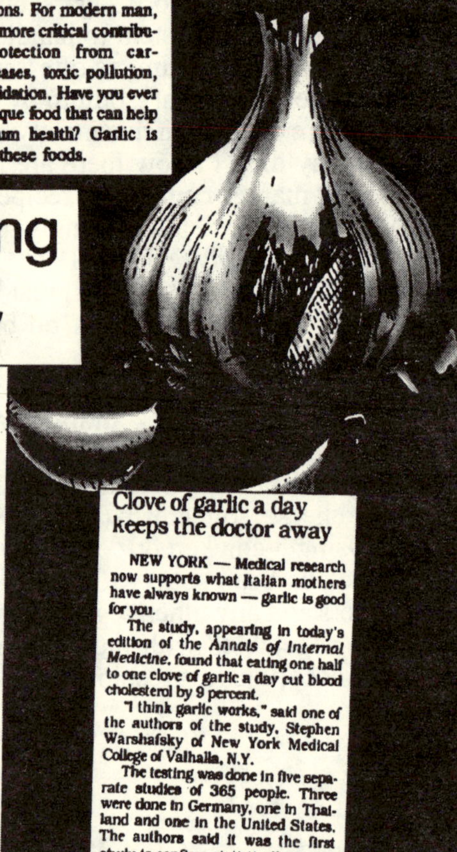

Garlic growing in popularity

Garlic is earning a stronger place in the garden.

There is a national Fresh Garlic Association, and a number of states have promotional organizations. Garlic is one of the oldest crops grown worldwide and long was considered a giver of health, protector from evil, and even an aphrodisiac. It is used to flavor and season many food products. In some countries, the green tops are used as well as the bulb cloves.

In mild regions, garlic is a perennial plant. It is frost-hardy, and a period of cold improves growth and clove formation.

In 1609, the following appeared in a publication called "The Englishman's Doctor":

"Garlic then have power to save from death; Bear with it though it make unsavory breath; And scorn not garlic like some that think; It only maketh man wink and drink and stink."

Clove of garlic a day keeps the doctor away

NEW YORK — Medical research now supports what Italian mothers have always known — garlic is good for you.

The study, appearing in today's edition of the *Annals of Internal Medicine*, found that eating one half to one clove of garlic a day cut blood cholesterol by 9 percent.

"I think garlic works," said one of the authors of the study, Stephen Warshafsky of New York Medical College of Valhalla, N.Y.

The testing was done in five separate studies of 365 people. Three were done in Germany, one in Thailand and one in the United States. The authors said it was the first study to confirm statistically garlic's beneficial role in lowering cholesterol, which can build up in blood vessels and contribute to heart disease.

CHAPTER TEN

GARLIC FOR HEALTH

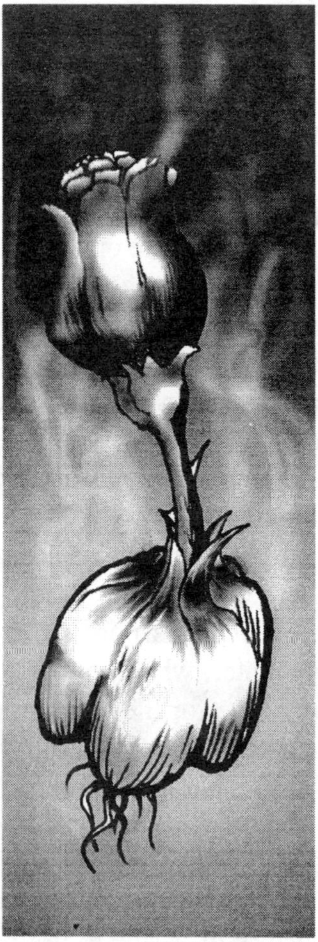

In a previous chapter was mentioned the low cardiovascular disease among Italians and other ethnic groups using olive oil as their principal oil in cooking. It is strange to me that very few writing about this fact never mention how garlic is also a prime condiment in all their cooking. Were you aware that true garlic lovers and users are a cult? (Joke!) If you are surprised by this statement, you should visit Gilroy, California, "The Garlic Capital of The World," as declared by *The Garlic Times*,[11] "The Newsletter of the Stinking Rose."© Surprised? Well, don't be, for, from ancient times, garlic has been idolized as a healing agent to the extent of having been found when archeologists opened King Tut's tomb. If you thought that all they found were those exquisite treasures of gold and precious jewels, you were sadly mistaken, for they also found—garlic! And why not? This truly versatile herb has been used throughout ancient times, in China also, as a cure for many of the diseases and complaints for which today's population is visiting the major clinics, doctor's offices and hospitals.

According to a recent newspaper article, the American Journal of Medicine reported upon a study at Tulane University School of Medicine, covering a 12-week period of 9 women and 11 men who took 900 mg of powdered garlic daily, in a control group of 14 women and 8 men taking placebo pills, all with cholesterol levels greater than 220 mg/dl. Choles-

and 8 men taking placebo pills, all with cholesterol levels greater than 220 mg/dl. Cholesterol levels dropped by 6% and low density lipoproteins dropped 11% in those subjects taking garlic pills.

A West German study published in 1990, enrolling 110 men and women with cholesterol levels between 200 and 300 mg/dl, reduced the cholesterol levels by 12% and the triglycerides by 17%, using 800 mg of powdered garlic each day for four months. (That's percent!)

My New England ancestral upbringing did not include any use of garlic, whatsoever, in cooking, or any other manner. As a matter of fact, there were only about a half-dozen families of Italian decent in my little home town, so I would say that we more or less "frowned upon" garlic and it's users. This seems tremendously funny to this author who buys garlic by the 3 to 5 pounds to grind in his cuisinart and freeze in jars. We keep one "working jar" handily in the refrigerator for daily use. Can't imagine being without it! I'm like the author of *The Book of Garlic*,[11] Lloyd J. Harris. I eat it "every chance I get!"

This book has been published for many years by Aris Books, Berkeley, CA. I've had my copy since my daughter, who knew of my love for the "stinking rose," bought me the book and a subscription to *The Garlic Times* back in the early 1980's. Filled with the serious history of garlic, to it's use as the "super herb," it's pleasures in cooking and related techniques, including recipes, they write about it's medicinal qualities, as do many prominent editorialists.

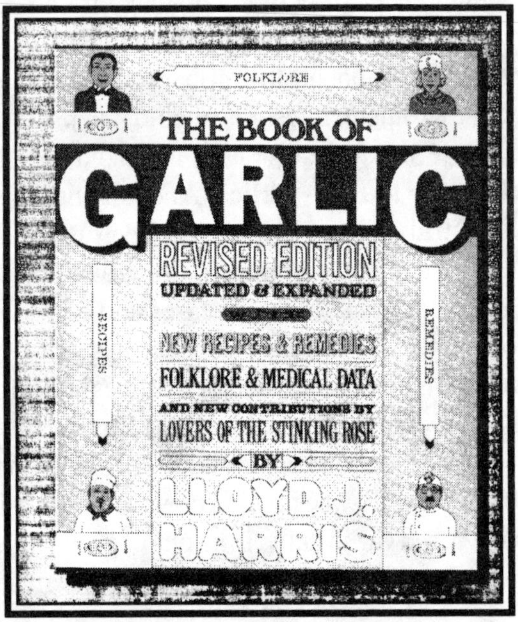

For instance, in *The Times*, "Garlic and Cholesterol, An Update From Rutgers University," indicates how researchers feel about the nutritional and medicinal value of this ancient herb.

The collection of articles I have in my "health library" cover the uses of garlic as ***preventive medicine***, in reduction of blood pressure; it's suspect as an inhibitor of cancerous tumors; warding off of the common cold (probably because no one can get that close to you!); and valuable as suggested remedies for 22 ailments from headaches to tumors, as noted in *The Codex Ebers*, an Egyptian papyrus from approximately 1550 BC. If you really want to follow previous use, you would have to read ancient history, covering the periods of Hippocrates, Aristotle, Mohammed and a Roman naturalist, Pliney the Elder, who touted garlic for 61 different maladies from hoarseness to hemorrhoids, which I would say covers a lot of bodily territory!

A more up-to-date study some years ago in the Readers Digest, by Bob Lin, PhD in biophysics and nuclear medicine at UCLA, post-doctorate at both California Institute and Massachusetts Institutes of Technology, credentials sufficient to write about most any food, not only the lowly, unsophisticated herb nick-named, "the stinking rose." Dr. Lin reviews garlic's potential medical contributions to protection from cardiovascular diseases, toxic pollution in the body and, due to it's richness in sulfhydryl compounds, garlic is a very effective free radical protectant. (These "free radicals" are the molecules which carry an extra electron as a result of our exposure to X-rays.)

His article is deeply technical but does outline the value of garlic as an immune stimulant as used in China in the 1970's; it's anti-inflammatory properties in injuries and rheumatoid arthritis; it's use on bacterial, fungal and yeast infections for thousands of years. And, believe it or not, garlic was used to prevent infections in wounds during World War I. (Penicillin must have been a blessing to later war wounded!)

Recently, while traveling in western Maryland, we encountered roasted garlic as a condiment served with hot rolls and butter. We did not actually recognize it until our daughter read to us from the latest copy of *Organic Gardening*, an article entitled, *Garlic:*

Still Healthy When Cooked.[12] (She did actually have the magazine with her!) It was great dinner conversation and related to the magazine having contacted a garlic researcher, Eric Block, PhD, University of New York at Albany, to learn that any dispute about the nutritional value being depleted by the roasting was to the contrary, for he stated that at least two of it's properties had been "bolstered" by the cooking process.

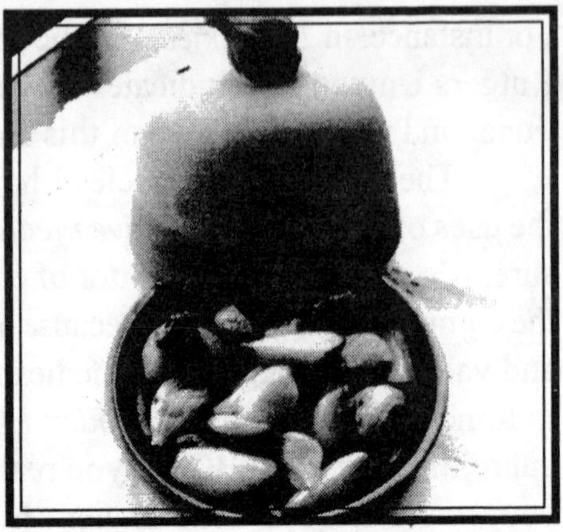

Furthermore, she read to us that, "the antibiotic compound within was diminished, but, the compounds that are believed to be effective against cancer were not affected by the cooking." In addition, the "stinking rose's" ability to inhibit blood clots and reduce fats in the blood stream was also enhanced. So, those who do not take to the raw taste of garlic may want to try roasting. I would advise the "elephant" variety for this tidbit of ***preventive medicine***. (Since that trip, we have been presented with a "garlic baker" which has enhanced our enjoyment of this herb as we spread the roasted product on crackers, hot rolls or "whatever."

Believe me, I have only touched upon the history and use of this ancient herb and recommend you buy either the book previously mentioned, or, *Garlic*, by Sue Kreitzman.[28] As you can perceive by the pounds I buy, I have found many personal uses for garlic and believe it to be very important in keeping my blood pressure under control, for I do have a family history of elevated pressure. When I really concentrate on doing so, I have been able to reduce my pressure by from 10 to 20 points. This entails a heavier than normal use and I would like to relate one of my personal "recipes" for use. This not only uses garlic, but lecithin and olive oil which you now know is believed to be most beneficial in circulatory disease control.

Mix... 1/2 cup cottage cheese (low-fat), 1 tbs lecithin, 1 tbs olive oil, 1 tsp apple cider vinegar, 1 (not scant) tsp crushed garlic. Add a bit of spice, such as basil, oregano and onion flakes to enhance the flavor.

Mix well and serve on crackers instead of eating that cholesterol-laded cheese for your afternoon or evening snack. Many times I fill a strip of celery with the mixture or toss some in my tossed salad or on sliced tomatoes instead of the usual mayonnaise. What's nice about this is that you are combining garlic with that other "miracle food," lecithin, helping and benefiting in your search for health and longevity through the medium of ***preventive medicine***. Don't think everyone agrees with my use of garlic in this manner, for I have a son-in-law who states that I have learned a new way to ruin cottage cheese, which he loves!

Quote: *Garlic! Thou art the supreme appetizer, the sole condiment, the glorious, the sovereign extract of the earth."*

Gustave Coquoit

And to add a bit of humor, a quote from a leading magazine I read recently:

"Scientists writing in the *Annals of Internal Medicine* report that eating garlic appears to offer tremendous benefits for your cardiopulmonary system. According to the article, eating half a clove of garlic will clear out your veins and arteries...and eating a full clove will clear out an entire movie theater!"

CAPITOL HILL UPDATE

After many years of patient waiting, the 10 year study ordered in April of 1982 and the five (5) year clinical trial results have been reported out this year.

The clinical studies (double blind) done by National Institute of Health (NIH) in the United States, the Netherlands and Israel were reported on at the Rheumatology convention in San Antonio, Texas, November 8th. With positive results being reported from all studies, we hope to see the intravenous clinical trials started promptly. After much work by Senators DeConcine and Harken and Congressmen Porter, money was appropriated in September 1992 for these trials. Barbara Matia, a long time supporter of Dr. Brown's work, tells us that in February it may again be necessary for all patients to remind our Congressmen we are anxious for the intravenous trials to begin. Barbara says she will keep us posted.

Arthritis breakthrough

A cure for arthritis?

Perhaps within two years, say British scientists, who have found a naturally occurring material they think prevents and cures rheumatoid arthritis. The material is "heat shock" proteins, obtained from heated blood plasma or from the blood of burn patients. Human tests and efforts to produce the proteins artificially are under way, says the head of Bristol University's Department of Pathology and Microbiology.

CHAPTER ELEVEN

ARTHRITIS RELIEF

Due to a few aches and pains prevalent a few years ago, diagnosed as "the beginning of **arthritis,**" I began gathering information relative to this most common of ailments. Rheumatoid arthritis being the most debilitating form of this disease, and, so far there has been very little research promising a potential cure. The best relief for years has been associated with aspirin prescribed in various formulas, but there are many so afflicted who have an allergic or other reaction to the use of aspirin. Tylenol, Ibuprofen and other pain killers are swallowed by the thousands, and, if you have never had this pain, it is almost impossible to realize the suffering which accompanies this condition.

In 1984 the *Washington Post*,[13] reported on the research and treatment results of Dr. Thomas McPherson Brown, who had great success in the use of tetracycline and IV's of other mycins as a powerful means of placing cases of rheumatiod arthritis into remission. *The Road Back*,[14] by Dr. Brown and medical writer, Henry Scammell, outlines Dr. Brown's years of research and successful treatment of thousands of sufferers throughout the United States. I do not use the word "sufferers" lightly, and neither will the reader who obtains and reads a copy of this book. It was not only written for public consumption, but also for doctors to learn and copy the treatment for their rhuematoid arthritis patients.

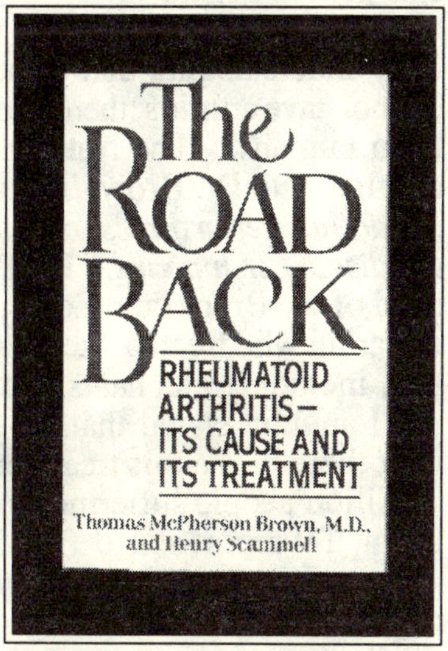

Similar to the previous mention of the Canadian medical group's treatment of the Doctors Shute for their "unorthodox" use of vitamin E in treating heart and cardiovascular conditions, Dr. Brown received the same verbal handling by his medical peers, who contended his treatment radical and unsuccessful. A careful reading of this book about the serious cases of rheumatoid arthritis put into remission, thereby allowing these previously and totally crippled patients to begin following a rather normal life, will convince even the worst skeptic of the value of Dr. Brown's lifetime of work. As stated by Dr. Brown, rhuematoid arthritis is ***"man's oldest affliction and has been with the human race longer than any other known disease."***

The *Post* also reported on Dr. Brown's treatment as administered to a gorilla, upon the request by officials of the National Zoo, Washington, DC. The gorilla was the only one born out of captivity 26 years before, and, from age 5 to age 26, was frail, having reached only 150 pounds total weight in his lifetime. The zoo director had decided to do away with this gorilla because he was so terribly ill with rheumatoid arthritis. Dr. Brown agreed to treat "Tomaka" with IV's of tetracycline which, over a three-year period, resulted in the gorilla's gaining strength and weight with progressively lessened intensity of attacks. At the time of the publication of *The Road Back,*[14] 20 years had elapsed and "Tomaka" was a healthy and an active **full-grown** gorilla!

Brown's theory was very basic from the standpoint of zoology, understanding that these animals in their natural environment did not have arthritis, therefore, it is a virus which the animals "caught" from humans. The National Arthritis Advisory Board (always in conflict with Dr. Brown's treatment) wrote, at that time, that *"gorillas do not get arthritis, and that rheumatoid arthritis refers only to the disease in humans."* Dr. Brown was backed in his theory by then head of the Brookfield Zoo in Chicago, Dr. Thomas Laughlin, a veterinarian who treated "very large" animals there and in private practice, including elephants, using Dr. Brown's method of treatment. Dr. Laughlin stated that he couldn't understand why the research isn't there to use this treatment on humans for there were more than 7 million people suffering from rheumatoid arthritis at that time. (A recent TV report stated 16 million so afflicted at the present time.)

Was Dr. Brown, author and co-author of nearly 100 articles relating to his research and treatment, a quack espousing a medical treatment unacceptable to the medical profession?

Though he was treated thusly by the medical profession, you be the judge, for his awards began with Phi Beta Kappa! A graduate of Johns Hopkins University Medical School, professor of medicine at the Rockefeller Institute in New York, World War II medical service, former Chief of Mt. Alto Veterans Administration Hospital in DC, 20 years with George Washington University Medical Center as Chief of Medicine, head of the Arthritis Institute in the National Hospital for Orthopedics and Rehabilitation in Arlington, VA. (and more). These are credentials worthy of recognition in the field of

AT THE CROSS ROADS TO THE ROAD BACK

Fifteen (15) years ago, knowing he was heading in the right direction Dr. Brown made an urgent appeal to all of his patients and friends for their essential support of the Thomas McPherson Brown Arthritis Institute in finding the cause and cure of rheumatoid diseases. The Thomas McPherson Brown Arthritis Institute's resulting efforts and publications, especially "The Road Back", obtained the attention of Congress who pushed the National Institutes of Health (NIH) into testing the tetracycline therapy.

The NIH and several participating clinics recently have found, 44 years later, that antibiotic (minocycline) therapy is safe and effective in treating rheumatoid arthritis. Despite this confirmation, many still have failed to recognize Dr. Brown's pioneering struggle that his many grateful patients and friends continue to support. Today, many doctors across the USA and the world still have not heard of or remain skeptical of tetracycline's benefits. The Thomas McPherson Brown Arthritis Institute's goal is to make the treatment known and available to the millions of arthritics who have not benefited. Thanks to Dr. Brown's efforts, the Thomas McPherson Brown Arthritis Institute has the critical data from his patients charts that show the benefits and safety of antibiotic treatment over a long period - unlike the currently used therapies. The arthritic patients should now be given the choice: to take the Road Back with antibiotic therapy or to continue down the road to disability and failure.

Even though Dr. Brown and his associates reported the first successful treatment of rheumatoid arthritis with Intravenous (I.V.) tetracycline in 1951. Only now, 44 years later, is NIH supporting a clinical trial of I.V. tetracycline. Hopefully the beneficial results of this clinical trial will be reported early next year (1996) without further delays.

From: THE SCANNER, winter 1995

medicine and his research should not be terminated nor abandoned.

Dr. Brown passed away in 1989, but during his lifetime he had established the Arlington Arthritis Institute. Those who were endeavoring to keep the clinic operating were increasingly inoperative due to age and were unable to continue their previous level of service. They worked diligently, and, with the help of the former medical director of the clinic, Dr. Cap Oliver, Mational Hospital for Orthopedics and Rehabilitation in Arlington, VA, they issued ***The Scanner*** shown above, as well as the bulletin entitled, ***FAIR***. Dr. Oliver was also directing The Arthritic Clinic of Northern Virginia. He has retired as of December 31, 1996, according to my report from ***The Road Back Foundation*** successor to the T. McP. Brown Arthritis Institute, which now seeks to continue this great study and treatment of rheumatoid arthritis. (See Appendix to this chapter). The author likes that name--***The Road Back Foundation*** for it perpetuates the name of Dr. Brown's book--***The Road Back.***

Many doctors throughout the United States were trained by Dr. Brown and his book outlines to physicians the dosage of tetracycline and other facets of his treatment. There are approximately 30 doctors and Rehabilitation, in Arlington, VA, who had been the T. McP. Brown Arthritis Institute Medical Director, and he advised that the National Institute of Health is now conducting some research on using tetracycline in treatment of arthritis. Dr. Oliver recently published an essay in *The Scanner,* published by the Institute, entitled, *Ongoing Treatment With Antibiotics,*[29] which outlines the treatment offered by the Arthritic Clinic of Northern Virginia in their "treatment of arthritis and musculoskeletal symptoms." When requesting a copy of the latest FAIR bulletin, ask for a copy of this also. (The Institute has limited means and would appreciate a small contribution and/or purchase of *The Road Back*—$17.00 including postage and handling.)

We hope that more doctors will learn the procedure and alleviate some of the suffering to millions afflicted with rheumatoid arthritis. I'm sure from my conversations with the Institute that they will be more than willing to aid one in finding medical help of this nature.

Ulcers are one of man's oldest diseases also. Perhaps the medical profession will not be as negative in the future relative to using an antibiotic to relieve rheumatoid arthritis. Medical research has now determined that bacteria has been the cause of peptic ulcers during all these years of suffering with same, and are now treating peptic ulcers with antibiotics!

Dr. Brown's Board of Directors was a "Who's Who" around the Washington, DC area, including United States Senators and Congressmen, some of whom had been treated by Dr. Brown, and whom also had obtained government research grants for the Institute. The famous novelist James Michener, was one of the approximately 10,000 treated by Dr. Brown. Mr. Michener related in one of his latest books that he was advised in his treatment for gout (a form of arthritis), not to eat certain foods nor drink red wine. Perhaps he received that advice from Dr. Brown.

The *American Legion Magazine*[15] recently reported on studies being conducted in the fight to cure this horrible disease. One avenue is from the genetic approach, that it is inherited and predisposes one to the disease. Research is endeavoring to develop a vaccine to prevent the disease from starting or progressing, but does state that "many years are needed to continue this research." These continuous studies are being conducted at leading universities and medical centers in Dallas, Chapel Hill, NC, Universities of Tennessee, Stanford, San Francisco, as well as the National Institute of Arthritis and Musculoskeletal and Skin Diseases in Bethesda, MD. Researchers are pursuing many paths to conquer this disease and feel that the attainment of this goal has never been so close. Let's hope so!

British scientists in the Bristol University's Department of Pathology and Microbiology recently reported to have found a naturally occuring material they think will prevent and cure rheumatoid arthritis. For a disease that has been with us almost since the "beginning of time," this is a new ***medical*** approach to this centuries-old disease. The material is "heat shock" proteins obtained from heating blood plasma, or, from the blood of burn patients. *"Perhaps within two years,"* say these researchers—and that is optimistic news! Let's hope it's not another of those premature announcements which give false hope to sufferers!

Why am I writing so much on this treatment? Because of the millions now suffering from arthritis. In addition, I feel that I was "touched" inadvertently by this use of a mycin when I had back spasms some years ago which I "cured" by falling to sleep with an icepack on my back. For the next four weeks I suffered severe arthritis in my hip, to the extent of having to use crutches for mobility. During this period, I became ill with a strep throat, which necessitated my visiting the emergency room of a local hospital where I had prescribed a mycin to be taken every 4 hours for 5 days. My throat was completely cured at the end of the medication period, but during that period, beginning with the second day, I began to feel relief in my hip condition and was completely cured of pain and walking freely without the crutches.

It was only a short time later that I read of Dr. Brown's treatment, prompting me to save the article with the firm intention of visiting with him and relating my experience, which, I'm sorry to say never occurred, for he passed away in 1989, leaving behind a lifetime of research benefiting mankind. As you can ascertain, however, great strides are being made in this search for a cure and I am even more optimistic after reading of the latest research

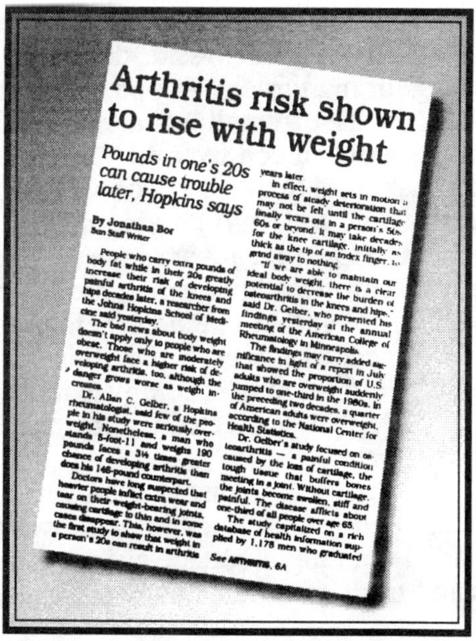

Arthritis risk shown to rise with weight

Pounds in one's 20s can cause trouble later, Hopkins says

By Jonathan Bor
Sun Staff Writer

People who carry extra pounds of body fat while in their 20s greatly increase their risk of developing painful arthritis of the knees and hips decades later, a researcher from the Johns Hopkins School of Medicine said yesterday.

The bad news about body weight doesn't apply only to people who are obese. Those who are moderately overweight face a higher risk of developing arthritis, too, although the danger grows worse as weight increases.

Dr. Allan C. Gelber, a Hopkins rheumatologist, said few of the people in his study were seriously overweight. Nonetheless, a man who stands 5-foot-11 and weighs 190 pounds faces a 3¼ times greater chance of developing arthritis than does his 148-pound counterpart.

Doctors have long suspected that heavier people inflict extra wear and tear on their weight-bearing joints, causing cartilage to thin and in some cases disappear. This, however, was the first study to show that weight in a person's 20s can result in arthritis years later.

In effect, weight sets in motion a process of steady deterioration that may not be felt until the cartilage finally wears out in a person's 50s, 60s or beyond. It may take decades for the knee cartilage, initially as thick as the tip of an index finger, to grind away to nothing.

"If we are able to maintain our ideal body weight, there is a clear potential to decrease the burden of osteoarthritis in the knees and hips," said Dr. Gelber, who presented his findings yesterday at the annual meeting of the American College of Rheumatology in Minneapolis.

The findings may carry added significance in light of a report in July that showed the proportion of U.S. adults who are overweight suddenly jumped to one-third in the 1980s. In the preceding two decades, a quarter of American adults were overweight, according to the National Center for Health Statistics.

Dr. Gelber's study focused on osteoarthritis — a painful condition caused by the loss of cartilage, the tough tissue that buffers bones meeting in a joint. Without cartilage, the joints become swollen, stiff and painful. The disease afflicts about one-third of all people over age 65.

The study capitalized on a rich database of health information supplied by 1,178 men who graduated

See ARTHRITIS, 6A

being reported upon by the Johns Hopkins School of Medicine. This study on over a thousand graduates during the period 1948 to 1964, relates arthritis to the weight of these individuals studied over this period of time.

We have all heard of treatment for arthritis with gold salts, cortisone and harsh drugs, all of which give only temporary relief and in many cases serious side effects. There are numerous books written on the subject, if any reader is interested in further study, two I am familiar with published by Keats Publishing Company, *Arthritis,*[16] by Langer, MD, and *Arthritis, Nutrition and Natural Therapy,*[16] by Wade. Another is by the well-known health writer, Dale Alexander, *Arthritis and Common Sense.* I only read a summary of this book but feel that I benefited from his recommended treatment of chronic arthritis, not rheumatoid, based upon the use of cod liver oil ("to oil the joints," his wording), which I found to be quite successful in relieving quite severe pain I was beginning to feel in my thumbs, shoulder and ankles.

His treatment of 1 tablespoon of cod liver oil, every other day for 6 months, then reduced to once per week, was given to his own mother successfully. Admittedly, cod liver oil has a noxious taste without mixing it with 2 ounces of whole milk (contains more fat) or fresh orange juice, not from concentrate. Also, there are two other facets of his treatment:

1. Take it on an empty stomach at least 4 hours after your last food;

2. Do not take any food for one hour after taking the mixture.

For goodness sake, don't take it straight (unless you're qualifying for martyrdom) or you will quit the treatment in a hurry!

I have a small jar holding 6 ounces of liquid, in which I put 5 tablespoons of cod liver oil and fill to nearly the top, leaving room for shaking. I found that two swallows took 1/5 of the mixture, thereby easily (and tastefully) giving me my one tablespoon each time. I take it before retiring or in the middle of the night, if awakened for any reason. One hour before breakfast is a good time to take same, if you can wait that one hour before eating, including of course, the recommended mixture by Dr. Rinse to round out your nutritious breakfast. I did get almost complete relief after the 6 months, and, being human, I then neglected the treatment until the pain once again reminded me.

In my last conversation with Dr. Rinse, he told me of a German Dr. Johanna Budwig, who was treating patients successfully with a mixture of cottage cheese and 10% raw linseed oil. I understand from conversations with Dr. Rinse that Dr. Budwig has also been using raw linseed (flaxseed) oil against cancer tumors with great success.

I am about to try the linseed oil for my minor arthritis, having just purchased the flaxseed oil, and hope that in addition to the cod liver oil treatment, I will benefit my skin as well as getting relief from the arthritis condition. I plan to use both twice per week, so hope someday I can report to you that I no longer suffer the pain of chronic arthritis and have noticeable improvement in my skin!

GOOD LUCK AND PLEASANT RELIEF!

Appendix:

On July 31, 1996, the Arthritis Institute founded by Dr. Brown closed its doors. The Institute board of directors voted to pass their ruling list on to the ***Road Back Foundation*** and to forward calls to the successor foundation so as to continue providing patients and supporters information on antibiotic therapy. The ***Road Back Foundation*** is a non-profit, volunteer, educational organization founded by patients who were treated successfully with antibiotics.

Concerned that information about antibiotic therapy would no longer be available unless they continued the effort, they organized for that purpose in October of 1992, were incorporated by the State of Ohio in January of 1993, and received their IRS tax exempt status in March of 1993. Since that time, they have reached many thousands of patients and physicians worldwide with their publications. Their quarterly publication ***The Intercessor***, is available by writing to:

The Road Back Foundation, 4985 N. Lake Hill Road,
Delaware, OH, 43015-9249

Tel. 614-881-5601

They publish a doctor information packet for patients and physicians which includes a protocol for this therapy developed from Dr. Brown's published works, patient case histories and summaries of scientific journal articles supporting his theory.

The Arthritis Clinic of Northern Virginia will be operating under a new director as of January 1, 1997.

Dr. Philip W. Kemp, 2465 Army Navy Drive
Arlington, VA 22206

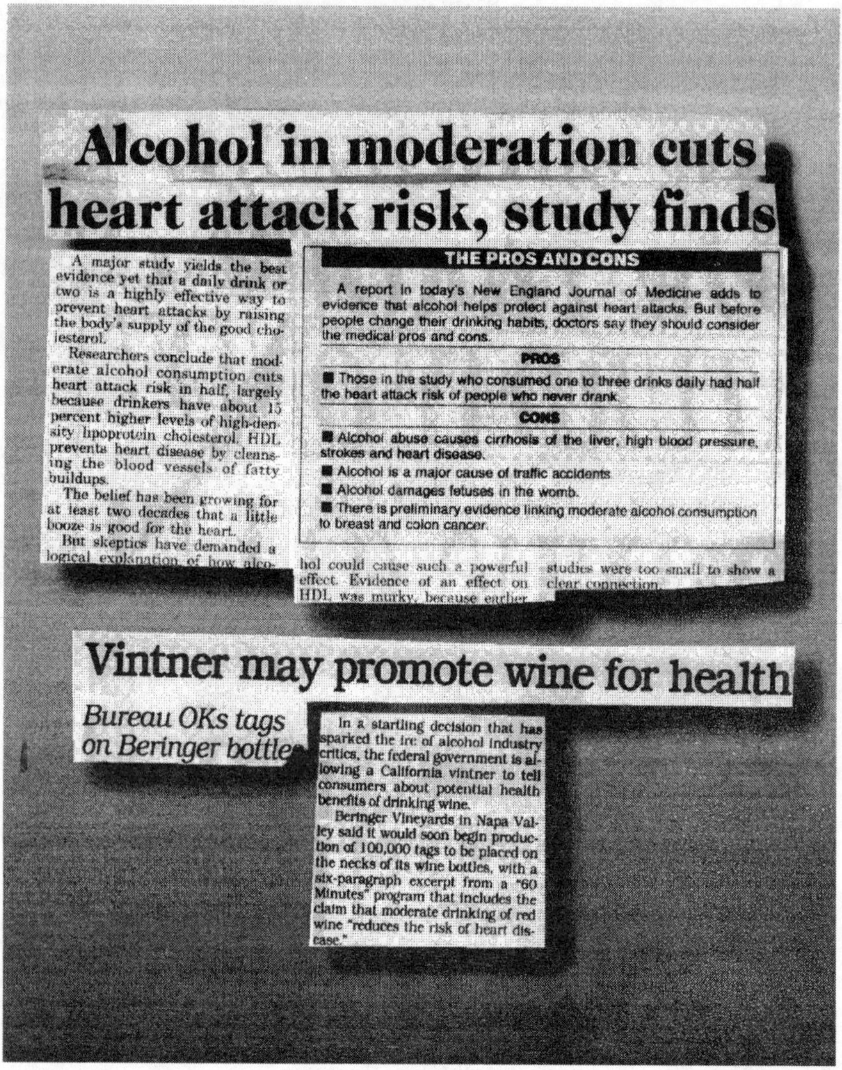

Alcohol in moderation cuts heart attack risk, study finds

A major study yields the best evidence yet that a daily drink or two is a highly effective way to prevent heart attacks by raising the body's supply of the good cholesterol.

Researchers conclude that moderate alcohol consumption cuts heart attack risk in half, largely because drinkers have about 15 percent higher levels of high-density lipoprotein cholesterol. HDL prevents heart disease by cleansing the blood vessels of fatty buildups.

The belief has been growing for at least two decades that a little booze is good for the heart.

But skeptics have demanded a logical explanation of how alcohol could cause such a powerful effect. Evidence of an effect on HDL was murky, because earlier studies were too small to show a clear connection.

THE PROS AND CONS

A report in today's New England Journal of Medicine adds to evidence that alcohol helps protect against heart attacks. But before people change their drinking habits, doctors say they should consider the medical pros and cons.

PROS

- Those in the study who consumed one to three drinks daily had half the heart attack risk of people who never drank.

CONS

- Alcohol abuse causes cirrhosis of the liver, high blood pressure, strokes and heart disease.
- Alcohol is a major cause of traffic accidents.
- Alcohol damages fetuses in the womb.
- There is preliminary evidence linking moderate alcohol consumption to breast and colon cancer.

Vintner may promote wine for health

Bureau OKs tags on Beringer bottles

In a startling decision that has sparked the ire of alcohol industry critics, the federal government is allowing a California vintner to tell consumers about potential health benefits of drinking wine.

Beringer Vineyards in Napa Valley said it would soon begin production of 100,000 tags to be placed on the necks of its wine bottles, with a six-paragraph excerpt from a "60 Minutes" program that includes the claim that moderate drinking of red wine "reduces the risk of heart disease."

CHAPTER TWELVE

WINE AS MEDICINE

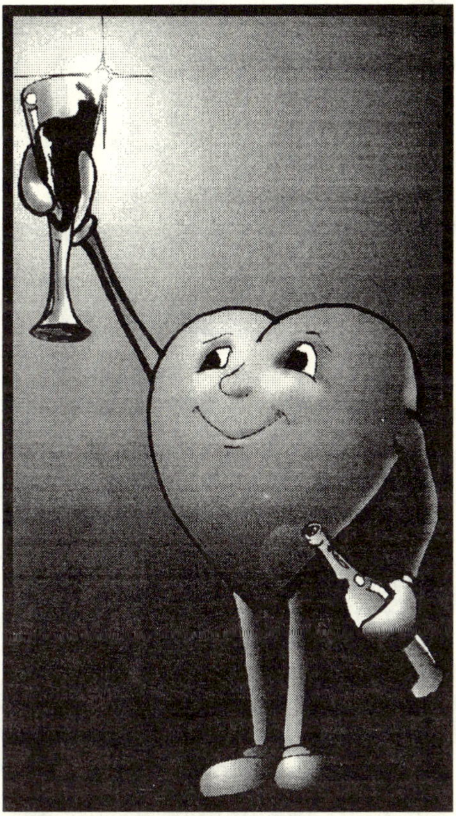

You have to understand that my life style and health allows the use of alcohol in moderation. As a matter of fact I had a bit of angina a few years ago (before heavy use of lecithin), and a doctor in the Boston clinic asked what I did for it. I told him I had a simple cure of one jigger of brandy or whiskey which relieved my angina in just a few minutes. He sort of nodded his head and prescribed nitroglycerin. I know that thousands of heart patients are helped by the use of nitroglycerin, but I became so dizzy it frightened me more than the angina, causing me to return to my "home-made" remedy. Upon moving to my present state, I located a heart specialist for examination purposes, who gave me a complete examination, including a stress test which I completed to his surprise with no sign of any serious defect- at age 75. I was honest with him and did relate my past history of angina and my "cure" or relief. He smiled and agreed that if it worked that was all that was necessary. However, when I related bouts of "shortness of breath" to him, he ordered tests which proved that my heart attack of nearly 38 years ago is now causing "functional" problems which he has controlled with medication. No more angina!

Some years back, I decided that I would like to make wine, similar to that which my dad's generation used to have "working" in the cellar. I had been working with a broker in western New

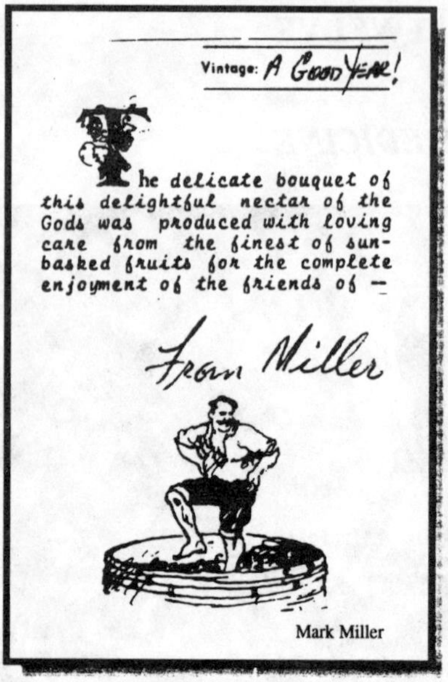
Vintage: A Good Year!
The delicate bouquet of this delightful nectar of the Gods was produced with loving care from the finest of sun-basked fruits for the complete enjoyment of the friends of —
From Miller
Mark Miller

York who took me to meet his father, then in his late 80's. As a token of hospitality, he went to his wine cellar (followed by me), drew a pitcher of wine from a barrel and I enjoyed a wonderful visit with this grand senior citizen. It was then that I made the decision to make my own wine, which I found to be an all-consuming avocation, never having realized the work involved doing it on a rather professional basis.

I was most fortunate in having been recommended to Mark Miller, author of, *Wine—A Gentleman's Game,*[17] at the very beginning of this wine-making venture. During our first meeting, he offered his jeep for transporting my newly purchased grapes to his winery, where he allowed me to use his equipment in the first stages of production, and from that time forward, gave me excellent professional guidance. I was amazed at his generosity but humbly advised by him that people who work in the wine industry are most cooperative and friendly, which I found to be true and our friendship continues to this day.

Mark is not just a winemaker, but semi-retired from his well-known illustration profession, his illustrations having appeared in magazines all over the world. Having spent many years in France where he obtained his wine interest, he returned to this country and built a very successful winery, promoting the first farm winery bill in America, in the State of New York, said bill now having been copied by many states nationwide. Mark also allowed me to use some of the illustrations for this chapter from his book. I invite those of you

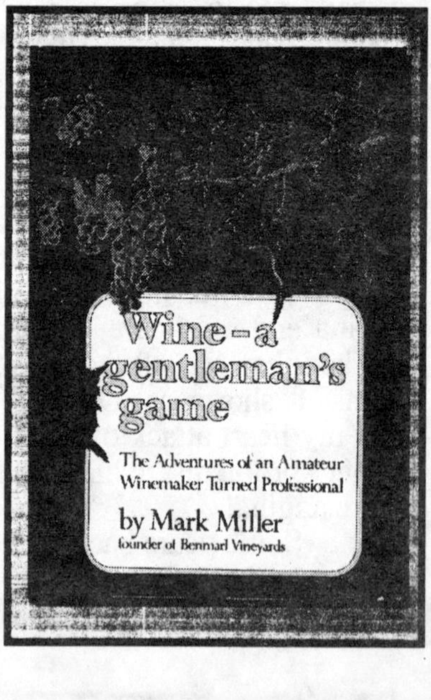

interested in wine and art to visit his "Gallery in the Winery," Benmarl Vineyards in Marlboro, N.Y.

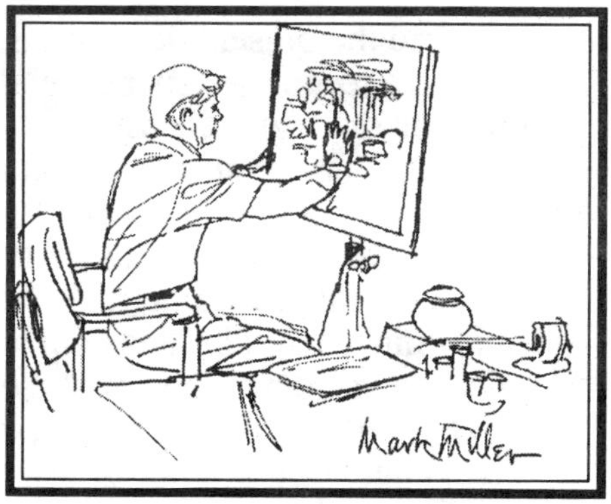

My interest in wine as ***preventive medicine*** led to the reading and study of many books on the subject, especially those relating to the healthful qualities of **red** wine when drunk in moderation. *Wine and Your Well-Being*[18] by Salvatore Pablo Lucia, MD, who was also the author of other books on the subject dating back to 1954. At the time of writing the above book, Dr. Lucia was Professor Emeritus of Medicine at the University of California School of Medicine in San Francisco. He had been on the faculty of the Medical School since 1931 and was also Chairman of the Department of Preventive Medicine.

The *Wellness Letter,* June 1993, answered a question in their "Ask The Experts" section, relative to **white** wine as beneficial to the heart. Their answer suggested that a couple glasses of white wine could also be beneficial to the heart, though they did note that drinkers preferring wine as their primary source of alcohol consumption did have less coronary artery disease. However, they did not rule out the possibility that wine drinkers as a group might also have a more healthful diet, and went on to remind the reader that heavy drinking of alcoholic beverages is a "good way to ***cause*** heart and liver disease, as well as more highway accidents!"

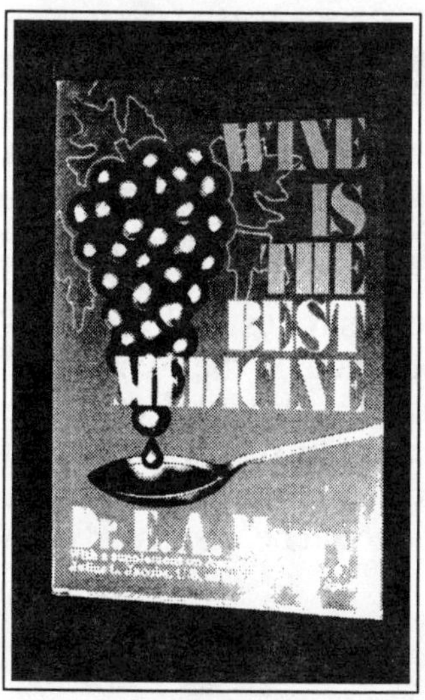

Another book, *Wine Is The Best Medicine,*[19] by Dr. E.A. Maury, was published in 1974. Dr. Maury was a general practitioner, an acupuncture specialist and a homeopathist, who claimed a high success rate among patients he had treated with red wine. The book was a best seller in Europe and one of ten other books he authored on various aspects of medicine. His book outlines the use and dosage he used for many conditions, including high cholesterol and atherosclerosis. (That was even before the present day concern about cholesterol.)

As a recent newspaper related, after the CBS "60 Minutes" program on drinking red wine,

"*It's nice to know that what you've been doing all along is healthy.*"

To carry the benefits of the consumption of red wine further, the Federal government has now given permission to a vintner in California to label bottles with an excerpt from the "60 Minutes" program, over tremendous public objections, I might add!

One of my client friends, when in business, was a widow who had angina. I told her of my relief method for my angina and suggested that she try a drink of sherry wine before retiring, but was advised that she wouldn't even give such a thing consideration due to her religious beliefs. I reminded her that the Bible says "*drink wine for one's infirmities,*" and that Christ's first miracle was the changing of water into wine at a wedding in Cana. Many of the English ladies of my heritage drank their tea at 4PM, but were also known to love their glass of sherry.

I'm not promoting alcoholism, or the promiscuous drinking of alcoholic beverages, by relating this event and the books that have been written on the subject, but just want to bring out the nutritional qualities found in wines as ***preventive medicine,*** and as outlined in these publications. In the event the reader is inclined towards same as a preventive measure, I must, however, add for you sufferers from gout, that red wine is a "no-no," from other studies I have read.

Though we have been concentrating on wine as preventive medicine in this chapter, I would like to call the reader's attention to a most recent *New England Journal of Medicine* (December 1993) article reporting on research done on alcohol in moderation as it cuts heart attack risks in half. Specifically stated-only a drink or two is recommended daily, which increases the HDL (high-density lipoproteins cholesterol) by 15%. They give the "pros" and "cons"-"pros" as mentioned above, and "cons" of the possibility of cirrhosis in some individuals, high blood pressure, strokes and heart disease, cause of traffic accidents, damage to fetus in the womb, all from the abuse of alcohol. They also warn of preliminary evidence of even moderate alcohol consumption being linked to breast and colon cancers. However, one of the medical researchers states, "the benefits have to outweigh the risks which should be discussed with your doctor."

I might add here those framed bible quotations hung at the entrance to my former wine cellar by an old neighbor and dear friend:

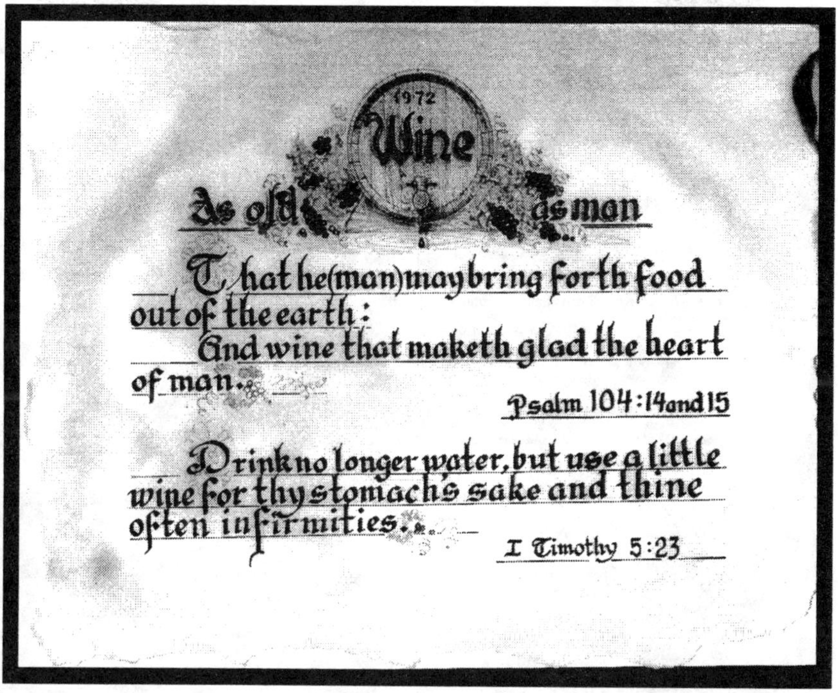

MONDAY May 16, 1994

Report attacks 'bad' fat

Says margarine may be a health bandit

Associated Press

WASHINGTON — A startling new report out of Harvard says a little-known type of fat that lurks in margarine and other processed foods could be responsible for 30,000 of the nation's annual heart disease deaths.

An article in today's American Journal of Public Health said the trans fatty acids found in those foods are probably worse than saturated fat. Margarine has long been touted as a healthy alternative to butter.

"Many people who are trying to make good nutritional decisions ... are being grossly misled," said Dr. Walter Willett, Harvard's nutrition chief.

But other scientists said Willett is overreacting.

"Yes, it's true they raise your cholesterol level but whether they're going to impart the same risk as saturated fat is still unknown," said Dr. Margo Denke of the University of Texas.

Doctors have long warned people to avoid saturated fat, the animal fat found in butter and meats, in favor of polyunsaturated vegetable oils, which do not pose a heart risk.

But liquid oils aren't always practical, so food manufacturers solidify them in a process called hydrogenation. Hydrogenated vegetable oils are used to make margarine and a wide range of cookies, crackers and other processed foods.

Hydrogenation creates a new type of fat called trans fat.

Don't pass the margarine: Its fat may be bad for you

Associated Press

WASHINGTON — A new report out of Harvard says a little-known type of fat that lurks in margarine and other processed foods could be responsible for 30,000 of the nation's annual deaths from heart disease.

U.S. researchers reported last year that diets high in margarine, long touted as a healthy alternative to butter, and similar foods could double the risk of heart attack.

But an article in today's *American Journal of Public Health* goes even further, saying that the trans fatty acids found in those foods are probably worse than saturated fat.

"Will people be shocked? I suspect so," said Dr. Walter Willett, Harvard's nutrition chief and a renowned researcher on diet and heart disease. "Many people who are trying to make good nutritional decisions for themselves and their kids are being grossly misled."

to avoid saturated fat, the animal fat found in butter and meats, in favor of polyunsaturated vegetable oils, which do not pose a heart risk.

But using liquid oils is not always practical, so food manufacturers solidify them in a process called hydrogenation. Hydrogenated or partially hydrogenated vegetable oils are used to make margarine, shortening and a wide range of cookies, crackers, chips and other processed foods.

Hydrogenation creates a new type of fat not found in nature; hence the name trans fat.

Studies show trans fats increase the so-called bad cholesterol — low-density lipoprotein, or LDL cholesterol — to the same degree that saturated fat does. But some studies show they also decrease good cholesterol — HDL or high-density lipoprotein.

And last spring, researchers reported that diets with lots of trans fats more than double Americans' risk of heart attack.

CHAPTER THIRTEEN

MISCELLANEOUS THOUGHTS

Throughout these writings I have continuously advised that one should be guided by the advice of one's physician, but, prompted by a recent newspaper editorial about the announced scientific breakthrough in research, I feel that it might be time herein to expand a bit on same. The announcement seemed promising in saving lives of those afflicted with certain diseases or conditions, such as high blood pressure and leukemia, continuing on to say that, "maybe" or "eventually," these medications will be available to cure such conditions-"in years to come."

There is a great necessity for researchers, doctors and those reporting journals, to insert disclaimers early in reporting these breakthroughs to lessen the heartbreak of those so afflicted with the condition mentioned. The medical discovery being reported upon may never prove to be effective or be a cure, at least not so in one's lifetime.

Even today, as I write, our newspapers and TV's are reporting on the merits of the drug, Tacrine, which was first introduced with great fanfare 6 years ago as a potential cure for alzheimers disease. The optimistic declarations have so far not lived up to expectations, dashing the hopes of so many people whose relatives are suffering from this affliction. It has shown to be effective on only 30% of the test cases and there is a side effect detrimental to the function of the kidneys, according to the reports. I think that this emphasizes the importance of early disclaimers or "softening" of the anticipated results of any new drug, even though future tests may prove to be more effective. (The newspaper editorial on the next page came into my possession just prior to publication of this book, so I am pleased to see that they are in agreement with me.)

The use of ingredients mentioned herein for many conditions are never offered as a cure for any ailment. There is no doubt that many people using them have been helped, including this writer, and relieved of some of the stress and pain accompanying certain conditions, but there are no medical cures as noted, nor miracle workings.

Through the years great strides have been made in medical research which have increased our life expectancy. Statistics are offered proving that less die or are crippled from heart attacks, polio and other diseases, causing us to believe that someday there will be no such diseases. We thought that tuberculosis was wiped out but we see a sudden recurrence, and, added to that is the horrible threat of AIDS, giving researchers another battle. A friend of mine is one of

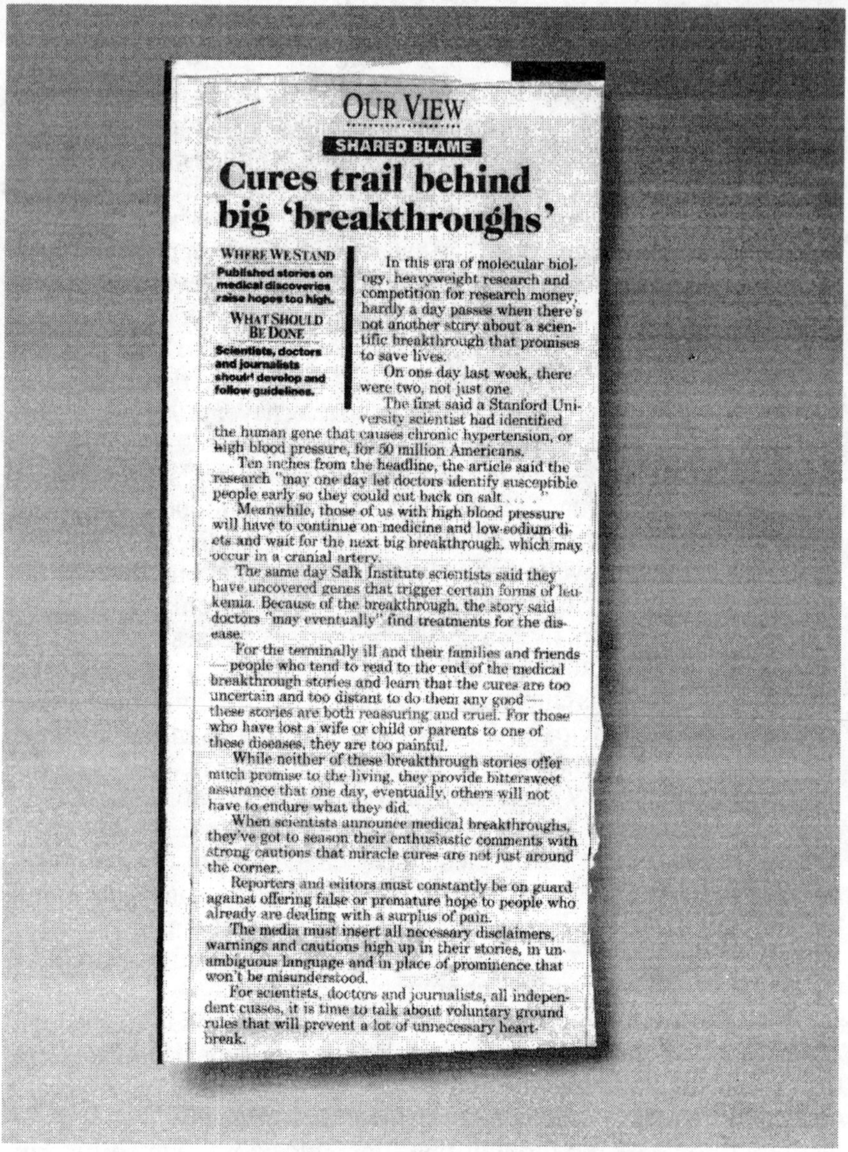

OUR VIEW

SHARED BLAME

Cures trail behind big 'breakthroughs'

WHERE WE STAND

Published stories on medical discoveries raise hopes too high.

WHAT SHOULD BE DONE

Scientists, doctors and journalists should develop and follow guidelines.

In this era of molecular biology, heavyweight research and competition for research money, hardly a day passes when there's not another story about a scientific breakthrough that promises to save lives.

On one day last week, there were two, not just one.

The first said a Stanford University scientist had identified the human gene that causes chronic hypertension, or high blood pressure, for 50 million Americans.

Ten inches from the headline, the article said the research "may one day let doctors identify susceptible people early so they could cut back on salt. . . ."

Meanwhile, those of us with high blood pressure will have to continue on medicine and low-sodium diets and wait for the next big breakthrough, which may occur in a cranial artery.

The same day Salk Institute scientists said they have uncovered genes that trigger certain forms of leukemia. Because of the breakthrough, the story said doctors "may eventually" find treatments for the disease.

For the terminally ill and their families and friends — people who tend to read to the end of the medical breakthrough stories and learn that the cures are too uncertain and too distant to do them any good — these stories are both reassuring and cruel. For those who have lost a wife or child or parents to one of these diseases, they are too painful.

While neither of these breakthrough stories offer much promise to the living, they provide bittersweet assurance that one day, eventually, others will not have to endure what they did.

When scientists announce medical breakthroughs, they've got to season their enthusiastic comments with strong cautions that miracle cures are not just around the corner.

Reporters and editors must constantly be on guard against offering false or premature hope to people who already are dealing with a surplus of pain.

The media must insert all necessary disclaimers, warnings and cautions high up in their stories, in unambiguous language and in place of prominence that won't be misunderstood.

For scientists, doctors and journalists, all independent cusses, it is time to talk about voluntary ground rules that will prevent a lot of unnecessary heartbreak.

By special permission of the News Journal Company, Wilmington, DE these government researchers on AIDS, giving me a first-hand look into the tremendous amount of work in which they are continually involved.Medical history is full of changes but very few cures, which is why so many of us are following the path of ***preventive medicine*** and sound nutrition, substituting foods we never dreamed would be the answer to our future health, such as soybeans, wheat germ, brewer's yeast, lecithin, beans, legumes and many more.

I'm reminded of a statement I heard many years ago, by a Japanese scientist. Quote: "*If one would drink one bottle of beer before retiring, one would have a day's supply of vitamin B, would sleep well and be relieved of any possible constipation.*" Of course, this is an alcoholic beverage and not considered necessary or permissible for medical or religious reasons by many people, but today, if one were so inclined, there is alcohol-free beer being manufactured.

My business travels throughout the State of New York and surrounding states, brought me into contact with most interesting people and their various diets in following the continuous search for health away from the fast foods of today. One such contact was with a couple, both with graduate degrees in agriculture, and ones who followed their studies into life. They were real nutritionists, conducting an agricultural radio program for their farm audience at 5AM each day-Ed and Bonnie Slusarzyk, of Utica, NY. Many mornings I would meet Ed at a local restaurant, the "Hungry" something or other, where he would pour that heavy cholesterol-laded cream into his coffee over my rousing condemnation, while he would reprimand me for adding "that chemical sweetener." However, I noted when lunching with both Bonnie, who did his scripts, and Ed, that they both ate from the "greens & grains," so I am sure that Ed dissolved that breakfast cholesterol satisfactorily. I still hear him on the air 20 years later as I tune in my radio at 5AM, using ear phones, so as not to awaken my wife!

Ed also had an interesting theory on hamburger which he purchased in 5-pound bags. Said he bought the meat of older dairy cows out of production and that the producers ground up the whole cow into hamburger-the filet mignon, rib roasts, etc., therefore, he was not eating the beef that most markets use for hamburger. His theory was, that from a nutritional standpoint, this was meat from animals having been fed the best of grains throughout their lifetime of milk production. The last contact I had with him was when he was in the middle of setting up a radio farm network in the northeastern U.S. His continued broadcasting 20 years later speaks for his continued good health, I would say. Perhaps if he reads this I will hear from him.

Some readers may criticize my mention of ground meat-hamburger—due to it's high fat content, and I will accept the criticism in relation to grams of fat being added to one's diet. Recent reports of the sad and tragic salmonella poisonings from having eaten hamburger which was poorly processed or refrigerated-and-under-cooked should be mentioned here as a warning to buy it fresh, refrigerate it and cook it suficiently to avoid serious comsequences. However, my information relative to high-cholesterol meats is that the cholesterol ingested from nutrients are not absorbed through the digestive tract, and also according to Dr. Rinse, even glands such as "sweetbreads," with high cholesterol content, do not increase blood cholesterol levels.

A young mother of my acquaintance many years ago refused to allow or feed her children any form of sugar or candy. They moved to California so I lost track of them for many years until the children had matured and were college graduates. When I next made contact, while visiting that section of the country some years later, I was not in the least surprised to learn that neither one of those children had ever had a tooth cavity! The young man stood at over 6 feet 6 inches and his sister nearly 6 feet. I don't have a feeling that they were deprived for not having had all the usual sugar in young diets. That was real ***preventive medicine!***

Perhaps it relates to one office manager I took to lunch when in business and he decided to have beef, because his religious beliefs were such that they never ate meat at home. He did state that about once a month he and his wife would have meat at home but did not give it to the children. I thought this strange and said so but he answered that the children didn't like meat because they had never had it. So perhaps it is similar to the above in not having had sugared products. It's all what we get used to in the diet so take my advice and get on the "band wagon" with those basic ingredients for a good breakfast.

Another business man whom I took to dinner one evening was a very religious young man who had also embraced vegetarianism as a way of life, to the extent that his wife was a bit critical. However, when we ordered dinner, he did not hesitate for a moment in ordering rib roast of beef, much to my surprise, which led me to speculate on his true dedication to a total vegetable diet-or-was it because I was paying the check? I'm not being critical but just wonder if some of these people find that there is a need for some other supplements added to the vegetarian diet. I'm sure that most vegetarians are sincere for I remember a vegetarian health food store in upstate New York where very tasty and nutritious dishes were prepared on the premises. I enjoyed a few of those preparations in my travels.

I have often thought of so many children going to school

with an empty stomach. The government and school systems have concentrated on lunches in the schools and perhaps they should do so on breakfast. Many states, including nearby Maryland, have adopted serving breakfast to children, thereby, hopefully, increasing their learning ability by substituting concentration on studies rather than their empty stomachs. As far as this author is concerned, this is a step in the right direction towards starting the day on a nutritional basis for these students.

I also noted recently that the school systems are allowing the fast food companies to supply the lunches in the school cafeterias, so question the level of nutrition they will be getting, especially the amount of fat grams per lunch. I'll probably get some flack from some of these companies, but advise you to read the fat content of these fast foods in *The Wellness Encyclopedia*[31] and judge for yourself the true content of these fast foods that our younger generation is devouring in great quantities.

However, my concern related to the high fat content of the "fast food menu" has been upheld by a 1993 survey conducted by the USDA on school lunches (whether by fast food operators or not). The USDA study of 545 schools surveyed offered lunches that exceeded the "fat target" for total fat consumption by 8% and twice the recommended level of sodium. **For the *$4.7 Billion* spent on this program annually, there certainly should be more attention paid to lowering the saturated fat content of these meals being served to our children.**

According to an Associated Press release to newspapers as late as June 1994, though the USDA is requiring school cafeterias to cut fat intake in lunches, ***the rule won't take effect until the school year 1998-1999***-two years to wait in improvement of our childrens' health! At least one school district is not waiting but have already changed their school menus--Fairfax County, VA, as mentioned in TV news coverage of this report.

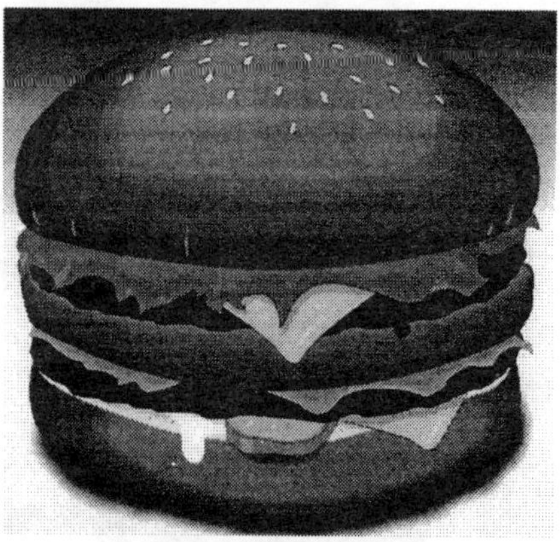

As one noted nutritionest stated, ***"Fast food is full of fat and preservatives—and expensive. You have to take food seriously—not just the nutrition, but the process."***

year 1998-1999-two years to wait in improvement of our childrens' health! At least one school district is not waiting but have already changed their school menus--Fairfax County, VA, as mentioned in TV news coverage of this report.

As one noted nutritionest stated, ***"Fast food is full of fat and preservatives—and expensive. You have to take food seriously—not just the nutrition, but the process."***

USDA Survey Shows School Lunches Are Still Failing to Make the Grade

Almost none of the public school lunch programs examined in a recent survey conformed to the Agriculture Department's dietary guidelines, and almost all provided far too much fat and salt, according to a USDA report released yesterday.

Rules requiring less fat in school food delayed

Associated Press

WASHINGTON — The government will require school cafeterias to cut the fat in lunches, but the rule won't take effect for four years.

That means a ninth-grader next fall will graduate from high school with the standard school fare, which has been found to provide as much as 38 percent of its calories from fat.

An Agriculture Department official confirmed yesterday that the deadline for requiring school lunches to meet the government's own nutritional guidelines won't be until the 1998-1999 school year.

That extended deadline provoked criticism from Public Voice, a consumer group that until 1993 had been run by Ellen Haas. Ms. Haas is the assistant secretary for Food and Consumer Services. She will announce the new proposals tomorrow.

"If that's the case then we think that that's unfortunate," said Tricia Obester, spokeswoman for the consumer group, which has long advocated an overhaul of the school lunch program. The group said schools could comply by 1995-1996.

Kevin Dando of the American School Food Service Association said the extended deadline "will help those schools that aren't as far along as they should be to meet these regulations."

The government's nutritional guidelines say people should get no more than 30 percent of their total daily calories from fat, and no more than 10 percent from saturated fat, the bad kind that can clog arteries and cause heart attacks.

The regulations to be announced tomorrow would require school lunches to fall within that range. School lunches already must provide one third of the recommended daily allowance for vitamins, minerals and other nutrients. To meet those goals, schools would no longer be bound by the current system of "meal patterns," requiring that all school lunches offer students one serving of meat or meat alternatives, two of fruit or vegetables, one of bread or grain, and milk, the official said.

The Agriculture Department will spend about $4.9 billion this year to serve 25 million children school lunches each day.

Baltimore Co. to start the day right

Schools to begin serving breakfast

CHAPTER FOURTEEN

"ORGANIC" and "NATURAL"

Variety-Balance-Moderation-the keys to one's **DIET.** To quote Hippocrates:

"Let Your Food Be Your Medicine;
Let Your Medicine Be Your Food."

My purpose herein has been to outline tidbits of my search for health through the years. I'm sure the reader will have ascertained that my path has been through the introduction of those nutritious foods designed to offset and prevent illness. I have admitted to the effects of stress and age on my body, but when I view many of my peers, comparing their health problems to any small ones affecting me, it is with a belief that I possess a rather vigorous old age due to my adoption of the three principles mentioned above, which include foods I have recommended within these pages.

As I write this, I have before me two excellent cook books on health which I will not name because so much has changed from a dietary standpoint since their publication. Hundreds of recipes, many using natural ingredients, are presented, and I suspect from my enjoyment of culinary repast that the end results of many of these recipes would be enjoyable. For instance, a fruit cake recipe with one full cup of butter. It is an accepted fact that we do try to forget about caloric consumption during the holidays when fruit cake is an old and popular delicacy, but what's the matter with using ground sunflower seed as the oil in this recipe? I have done so many times, following a very similar recipe, adding wheat germ, lecithin and brewer's yeast, along with all the spices, unsulphured molasses, honey or fruit juices as the sweeteners. Delicious!

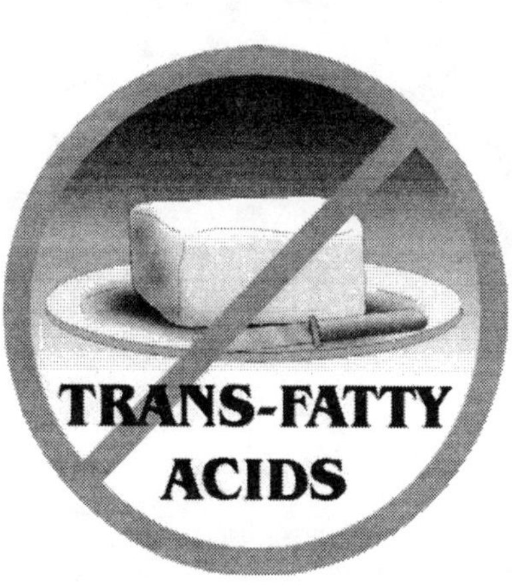

Butter is another casualty of the "cholesterol scare," having been eliminated from many diets. It is an excellent food, quite low in cholesterol content and containing short-chain fatty acid radicals, not the trans fatty acid used in marga-

What's 'Natural'?

Not-So-Natural Foods

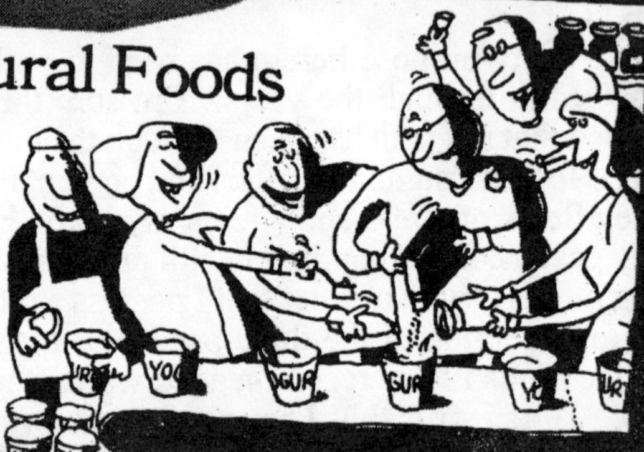

Natural foods have gone big time. The movement into the mainstream may have begun when the first spoon of sugar was attached to the first cold cereal, but it was probably the first spoon of grape jelly put into a carton of plain yogurt that marked the beginning of the end of natural foods.

When plain yogurt became fruit-flavored yogurt no one realized what the mainstreaming of natural foods would mean. They were soon to find out, as yogurt went on to bigger, though arguably not better, things. Some yogurts were frozen and turned into "healthy" alternatives to ice cream, but in fact many contain more calories than ice cream. Yogurt now has the distinction of having been the first junk health food.

Not everything in health-food stores is healthful, so check the labels carefully.

While there is no universal definition of "natural" produce, Maine, Oregon, Washington, California and Minnesota have set their own standards. Tom Harding, president of the Organic Foods Production Association of North America in Wind Gap, Pa., said those states regulate the growing and marketing of naturally grown produce, allowing farmers to label produce "natural" or "organic" only if they have limited their use of chemicals to those on an approved list.

rine to harden it. According to chemical research, this trans fatty acid remains in the blood and does not pass through the arterial membranes. For this author who has never eliminated butter from his diet, there can be no better taste on an ear of corn or in my vegetables! In moderation, of course!

The recipes for soups mentioned in one cookbook contain bacon, salt pork and ham, with no mention of removing the high cholesterol-laden fat (grease) prior to consumption, which doesn't surprise me, having lived through that period and observing the high rates of cardiovascular disease. During my college days at Maine, I visited the home of my roommate many times. I remember how his mother baked beans without salt pork, as well as the organic garden beside their house in Bucksport. They were in their 70's then and still living 20 years later when I revisited the area.

The author's information on trans-fatty acids in margarines and other foods came from my research material and my conversations with Dr. Rinse. It would seem now, according to this latest information being reported in newspapers, that Dr. Rinse and other researchers were convinced years ago that margarine was not the healthy substitute for butter we were being told by manufacturers and some nutritionists!

Our method of making stock from beef and/or bones, chicken, ham or ham hocks, leaving the fat and skin on while simmering many hours, was to strain and cool after simmering so that the fat can be discarded when solidified, and the meat portion saved for your soup. In addition, when simmering this stock, we have added all the vegetable peelings from carrots and potatoes, tops of celery, outside portion of the onions usually thrown away, stems from broccoli, cabbage and any other vegetable remnant which had been carefully stored in a plastic bag in the freezer.

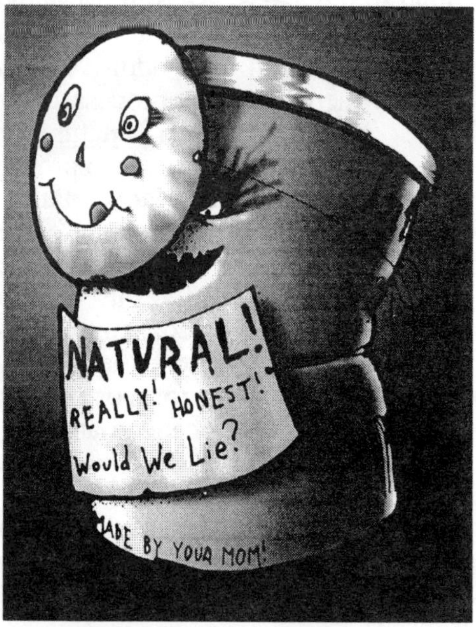
NATURAL!
REALLY! HONEST!
Would We Lie?
MADE BY YOUR MOM!

We don't just buy meat bones for soup, but save from previous meals and the trimming of the meats, all of which go into the "stock bag" in the freezer. It may sound complicated but really is simple and just a habit which you form while working around the kitchen. You could consider this a part of your conservation and environmental effort, thereby improving the environment while you are improving your health through a system of ***preventive medicine.***

Following the simmering process, you now have delicious stock rich in vitamins and minerals to be used for soup, sauces, greaseless gravies—whatever. If you follow this procedure, keep some stock in one-cup containers in the freezer for immediate use in preparing delicious dishes and your family and friends will wonder why your preparations taste so much better than theirs. Use the stock to cook rice and other vegetables to give an added touch.

One cookbook has page after page of organ food recipes, liver, kidneys, brains, tripe—all high cholesterol— foods which I used to enjoy until realizing the hazard of introducing all that LDL (low density lipoproteins) into my system, as well as the possible cause of my slight gout condition. If you've ever had a gout attack, which I don't wish upon anyone, you will know the all-consuming pain best described in one of James Michener's latest books.

The two cookbooks I have been discussing above both contain in their titles the words natural and organic. In today's market place these words are designed to create the impression that the foods being described are wholly nutritious and free from all chemicals. One of these so-called natural foods is a group of yogurt products found in the dairy case of most markets, sugared, flavored and frozen into what I would describe as a "not so natural" junk food after the addition of all these additives. I don't mean to pick on just one food for there are many processed similarly.

Any food grown is natural and organic, but, the method of growth and use of chemicals to promote growth is most important in the end product, for all plants retain a percentage of these chemicals when harvested. If your search for health is to follow the path of no chemicals, then look for that on the label of what you are purchasing, including the preservatives used in the processing.

This will be a constant battle on your part in your pursuit of health, but you can win the battle by not buying that which is "chemicalized" in one form or another. Note how many of those old favorite foods have changed and are now free of preservatives, all due to the watchful eyes of those of us who are concerned about our health.

You are the consumer, and, when you don't purchase the product, the processor and manufacturer will get the message and change or go out of business!

The word organic when used on labels could also be misleading because all multiple carbon compounds are organic according to legal definition. (Glad I took organic chemistry when at the University of Maine!) Flour is organic, but, if you read the Federal Register Standard Chemicals allowed in the bleaching and aging of white flour used in bread making, you would be frightened.

There are 1000 additives on the market used in foods we buy, some of which are a potentially hazardous chemical formula, either foreign to the body or not easily decomposed in digestion.

I'm delighted to hear that the USDA is finally demanding "true" nutritional labeling of all food products, with the words, natural, organic, lite, etc. having a standard definition. (The new USDA nutrition label included herein.)

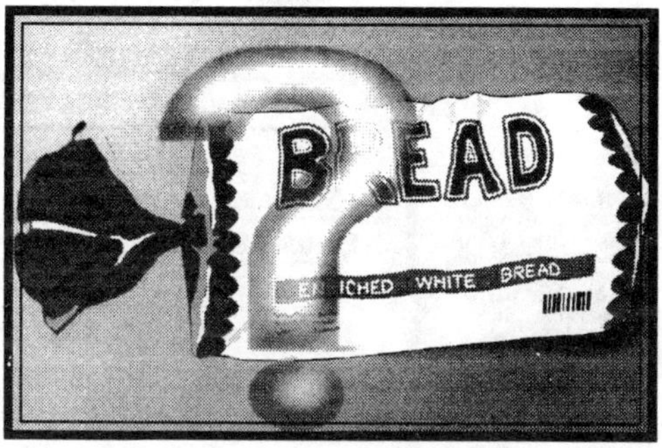

All together there are 93 additives allowed in the processing of flour and none have to be declared on the label! The same goes for whole wheat bread. This is not a war on the bread-making industry, but just a warning to you to carefully read the label before buying, for there are some very good breads on the market, minus chemicals and preservatives. These breads are a result of researchers and consumers endeavoring to protect the health of the buying public—***PREVENTIVE MEDICINE!***

Nutrition Facts

Serving sizes and nutrition facts show amount of daily requirements one receives from a serving size measured in metric as well.

Serving Size ½ cup (114g)
Servings Per Container 4

Calories of each serving size help one to regulate dietary intake which can be adjusted to meet each one's requirement.

Amount Per Serving

Calories 260 Calories from Fat 120

	% Daily Value*
Total Fat 13g	**20%**
Saturated Fat 5g	**25%**
Cholesterol 30mg	**10%**
Sodium 660mg	**28%**
Total Carbohydrate 31g	**11%**
Dietary Fiber 0g	**0%**
Sugars 5g	
Protein 5g	

List of nutrients and daily value provides a daily guide to nutrition and percentage of RDA per serving, plus guide to **fat**, fiber and sugar content. One can adjust serving size to provide more or less vitamin, sugar and **fat** content.

Vitamin and mineral content as a percentage of one's daily requirement based on an average of a 2000-calorie-per-day diet.

Vitamin A	4%	•	Vitamin C	2%
Calcium	15%	•	Iron	4%

* Percent Daily Values are based on a 2,000-calorie diet. Your daily values may be higher or lower depending on your calorie needs:

	Calories	2,000	2,500
Total Fat	Less than	65g	80g
Sat Fat	Less than	20g	25g
Cholesterol	Less than	300mg	300mg
Sodium	Less than	2,400mg	2,400mg
Total Carbohydrate		300g	375g
Dietary Fiber		25g	30g

Shows maximum fat and saturated fat, fiber, cholesterol and sodium levels of certain nutrients required for good health on approximately 2000-calorie-per-day diet.

Calories per gram:
Fat 9 • Carbohydrate 4 • Protein 4

Calories per gram of fat, carbohydrate and protein. Voluntary on most labels.

CHAPTER FIFTEEN

THE PROSTATE

I have concerned myself with prostate cancer since reading, *The Prostate,*[20] by J.I. Rodale (1967). Some years later when I was living in the Hudson Valley area of New York State, a newspaper article caught my eye when citing statistics from a local hospital, showing that the valley area had one of the largest percentages of prostate cancer in the nation. It was blamed upon the fact that a certain large national industry in upstate New York had for years been discharging PCB'S (polychlorinated biphenyls) from their manufacturing process, into the upper Hudson River, which was then, and now, the area's source of drinking water. There has been a serious effort to clean up the pollution in the river these past 20 or more years, but, this has not diminished the contamination caused by PCB's because they are settled into the river bed and can only be removed by dredging, from Albany down to New York City, a distance of approximately 150 miles. This will probably never be accomplished due to the high cost of such a project, and, if it was done, where would the sludge be deposited as waste for it will always be contaminated with PCB's!

During the ensuing years I have had friends and relatives afflicted by this insidious condition, some of whom have died a most painful death. There are approximately 34,000 men who die each year from this disease which makes it the second leading cancer killer of men—lung cancer being number one. In earlier studies, there was no comparison of ethnic groups. However, my research in library medical journals show statistics which should be of especial interest to blacks who have a much greater incidence of prostate cancer than whites. I was surprised to learn that Asians have no prostate cancer. We can't be sure why the incidence is greater among blacks

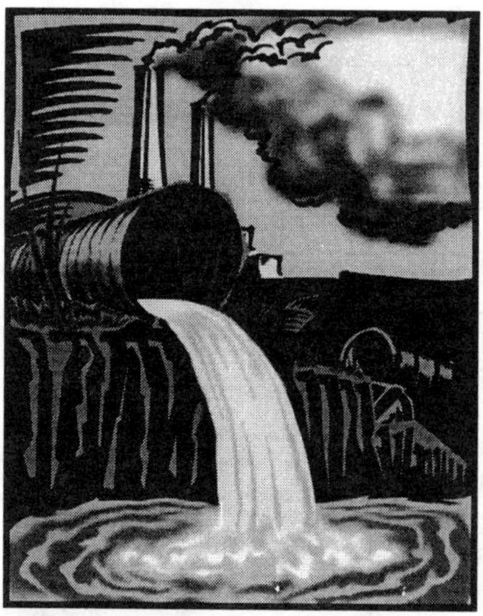

unless it's due to a higher fat diet. The Asians eat a healthy diet predominately of rice, which might account for their practically non-existent prostate cancer. (Perhaps this author will have to "eat his words" about rice consumption mentioned in Chapter Four!)

It would be interesting to see a study of Asian-American statistics on prostate cancer now that they are adopting a diet similar to our own. Europeans, who have had a low incidence of cardiovascular disease attributed to their high consumption of olive oil and red wine, might see the incidence of cardiovascular disease multiply, which could also happen to Asian-Americans being afflicted to prostate cancer in the future, both due to the adoption of the American diet.

Prostate cancer will afflict one in eleven men, and one out of three over age 50. Those are frightening statistics to we men, so now you understand my concern and reason for inclusion herein. Furthermore, the purpose of this book is to provide ***preventive medicine*** techniques through diet, including that which might benefit the male reader.

The surgical procedure during the past 25 years, since the Rodale book was published, has changed from a radical approach to a more simple operation. I do not intend to elaborate on the function of the prostate but only discuss the dietary means used in the past to alleviate the condition then and in the present. From a dietary standpoint, there hasn't been much change.

Over 40 years ago, Herbert Kenyon, MD wrote, *The Prostate Gland*[21] (1950), in which he analyzed the nutrients the prostate supplies to the sperm. It is basically similar to an egg in it's large content of the protein albumin--and--**lecithin**. We've covered that material pretty well, I'd say, and here it "pops up" again in another *old* study! Other investigators back in those years found substantial amounts of **vitamins A and C** in the sperm, both of which are prime fighters against infection, and the minerals **zinc** and **magnesium** are also present in unusual concentration. One could assume then that a prostate condition could probably begin with the lack of these vitamins A and C, and the minerals zinc and magnesium in one's diet. So, why not concentrate on supplying

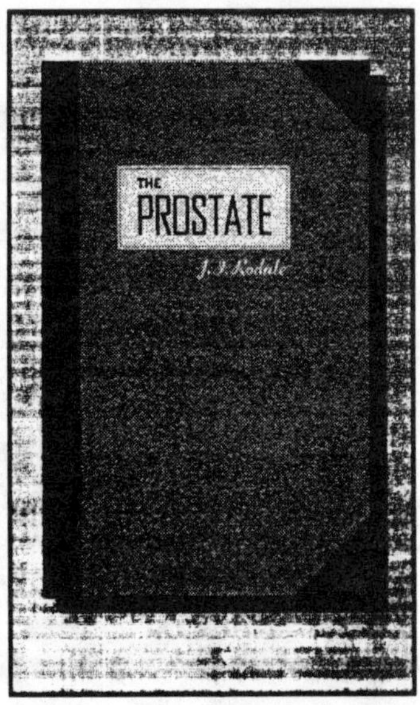

same to your body while you are healthy? ***Preventive medicine*!** A nutritional approach to this frightening disease.

However, my urologist reminded me, after reading this chapter, that, "one can not assume anything without scientific proof to support it, and there is none." I can understand his feeling and respect his professional opinion, but, the fact that doctors treating their patients with prostate conditions, using a nutritional approach in past years, though they were not professional researchers, does not mean that the results of their work were not valuable and effective. Years ago, according to Rodale, Dr's. James Pirie Hart and William LeGrande Cooper, of LosAngeles, kept detailed case histories of patients they treated successfully with tablets containing linoleic and archidonic acid. The oils and lecithin mentioned herein contain those acids, also referred to as vitamin F in the Rodale book.

I'm reminded of a friend in his middle 70's, diagnosed with prostatitis. The doctor advised surgery but my friend resisted due to his religious belief, being a Christian Scientist. However, when struck with a more serious attack a few weeks later, he agreed to the surgery, with the comment to me that, *"It's against everything I believe in."* For his family's sake, and he did have a young family due to a second marriage, thank God he listened, for the operation was a complete success.

Prostate cancer in men is likened to breast cancer in women, from it's high occurance and seriousness which can result in death. In the past, published facts about breast cancer clearly state that it might be genetic and occurs along family lines, but recent reports disagree with this premise. I believe prostate cancer and problems related thereto can be a nutritional deficiency as well as being caused by outside means, and probably more common in males who are less mobile in their work and lack good daily exercise.

My nutritional advice on this potential threat to the male reader (or the spouse who regulates his diet), as well as on other cardiovascular conditions mentioned within the confines of this book, is to closely analyze the vitamin and mineral tables presented herein, noting the availability of ***zinc*** and ***magnesium*** contained in wheat germ, brewer's yeast and lecithin, all contained in the basic breakfast containing these ingredients. When the lecithin is combined with the oil in the sunflower seeds, one's digestive system obtains the valuable fatty acid contained in the lecithin which is also necessary in the fight against prostate cancer.

Once again, my doctor noted that there is, "absolutely no evidence to support this statement," but the treatments and records kept by these older doctors, as mentioned above, seem to recommend lecithin and it's linoleate fatty acid as their primary treatment. In Dr. Rinse's research on the use of linoleate lecithin for atherosclerosis, his studies indicated that other credits mentioned in his book, *The Rinse Formula,*[5] outlined **extensive research showing reduced cancer incidence and tumor growth as a result of a diet rich in lecithin.**

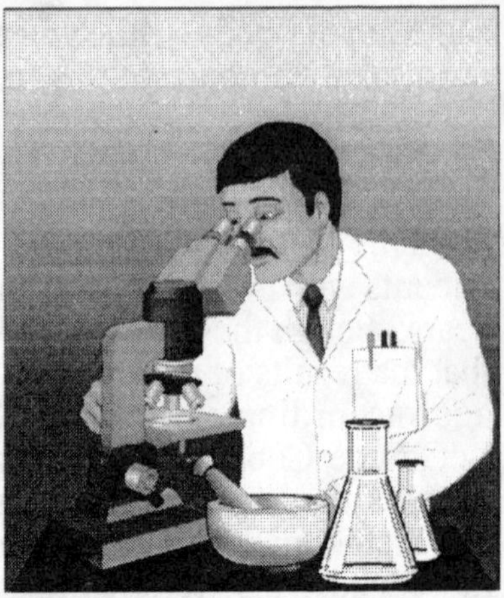

The addition to your diet of the other necessary vitamins A and C is simple by "popping a couple pills" daily-or-more sensibly, following a good well-rounded diet as recommended in these pages. Also, a great source of these minerals is in pumpkin seeds available to you in your health food store. Try chewing on a bit of parsley too for a good source of vitamin A.

What I haven't revealed to you from my study of this subject, is that all the recommendations here are contrary to the common practice of most diets, especially at breakfast when great amounts of products containing refined sugar, white (bleached) flour and high cholesterol-laded meats are consumed in the typical American diet. And I do hope that I have convinced the reader of the necessity of changing to a healthy and more nutritious breakfast. If you insist upon skipping a meal, do so at lunch, or, cut down on both lunch and that BIG dinner at night!

The State of Maryland has recently announced a campaign to eliminate prostate cancer through screening and testing. This will certainly be a worthy effort but will it ***prevent*** this serious threat of prostate cancer in the future? According to the article, Maryland is number six in the nation in lung, colon, breast and prostate cancer. (My doctor's statistics state that Maryland is second only to the District of Columbia, and that our State of Delaware is number three.) Staggering statistics and conducive to one's determination to fight the potential threat through ***preventive medicine*** as outlined by the researchers (right there in Maryland at the Johns Hopkins University Hospital Research Center), advising the eating of those vegetables containing **sulphoraphane.** Whether Maryland is number two or six in the nation, for your potential future good health, study Chapter 4 again. Where does your state stand?

If you are male-and-especially over age 50, by all means visit a urologist for a check-up before it's too late. I'm sure you've seen

Steve Allen on TV advising how he "beat" prostate cancer by early detection and was treated successfully. Detection is most important and a standard rectal examination has been the usual method of detection until recently.

Today, a new method of detection is a blood test, PSA-prostate specific antigen, usually given by a urologist (and now under question as to it's effectiveness). Any suspicion of cancer will result in the doctor taking a biopsy for positive determination. Though your PSA test does prove positive, according to Massachusetts General Hospital in a 1994 statement, you don't have to be rushed into a decision to operate. However, some of these tumors are very serious, but many are slow-growing and may never be life-threatening. They recommend an approach called "outcome analysis," using interactive videos to aid patients treatment decisions on benign prostate disease (or tumors). This video was developed by the Federation for Informed Medical Decision Making, Hanover, NH. Perhaps a reader might want to follow this avenue in the event of having been diagnosed as positive.

The American Cancer Society predicted 200,000 new cases would be identified in 1994, **double the 1980 figure**, with the principal increase in the 70 to 75 years and above age group. (This does not mean that younger men should ignore the PSA test or the local free screening tests being given, for all age groups show an increase).

Doctors see hope in new prostate cancer approach

By DIANA K. SUGG
The Baltimore Sun

BALTIMORE — In a novel approach to treating cancer, Johns Hopkins researchers plan to begin using prostate cancer patients' own tumor cells — and gene therapy — to enable the men's immune systems to kill the cancer.

The treatment, involving a complicated form of genetic manipulation, has been proven to work in animals with prostate and kidney cancers. And researchers believe it could be effective against other malignancies, such as colon cancer and melanoma. The treatment might even offer the patient a kind of vaccination to ward off future attacks by that specific type of cancer.

The U.S. Food and Drug Administration recently approved human trials of the therapy for prostate cancer, and Hopkins researchers plan to enroll eight patients in the next several weeks, a Johns Hopkins spokeswoman said Monday. Approval of the prostate cancer trial became public this weekend at a New Orleans conference for science writers.

About 40,400 men are expected to die this year from prostate cancer, the second most common cause of cancer death in men.

Hopkins researchers are already testing the method with a group of kidney cancer patients. Those results will not be made public until later this spring.

Experts say this type of therapy offers promise, particularly in cases where pieces of a tumor break off and travel through the body, spreading the cancer. Essentially, the therapy would train a person's immune system to seek out and destroy those small pieces — possibly for a lifetime.

To do that, doctors remove cancer cells from the patient's tumor and then insert into those cells a copy of a gene that stimulates the immune system. The cells are next irradiated, so they won't multiply, and injected back into the patient. Theoretically, the introduction of the genetically altered cells activates the patient's immune system to kill the cancer. The process takes several weeks.

"This is one of those things that is very exciting. It has the potential of being very significant, and it's something that I really think we have to try," said Dr. Otis Brawley, a prostate cancer specialist at the National Cancer Institute who is familiar with the Hopkins research.

Even so, researchers cautioned that the treatment is experimental and the studies are in preliminary stages. The therapy is not available to the general public.

CHAPTER SIXTEEN

"FOOD" FOR THOUGHT

I have endeavored to keep this book brief and present ideas of ***preventive medicine*** which I feel would be beneficial to the reader's health. There are so many facets to cover in writing any kind of health guide, and, if I tried to cover all I have available, I could fill as many pages as the latest food encyclopedia and bore the reader to tears. I have tried to present a very basic health formula as briefly as possible and let the reader make the decision on whether or not the adoption of my regimen would be beneficial and healthful to their well being.

The Encyclopedia of Food and Food Production and the Reader's Digest *Eat Better, Live Better,*[3] the first with 2322 pages and the latter with over 400 pages, when "digested," prove the theory presented here that variety in foods obtained for their nutritional value is certainly the path to follow for continued health and longevity.

The author is also pleased to note that in the nutritional recommendations contained in these two volumes they embrace and parallel the foods we mention as a basic and truly balanced, nutritional diet. The green vegetables, whole grains, nuts, beans, peas and legumes will lead you down the path of good health.

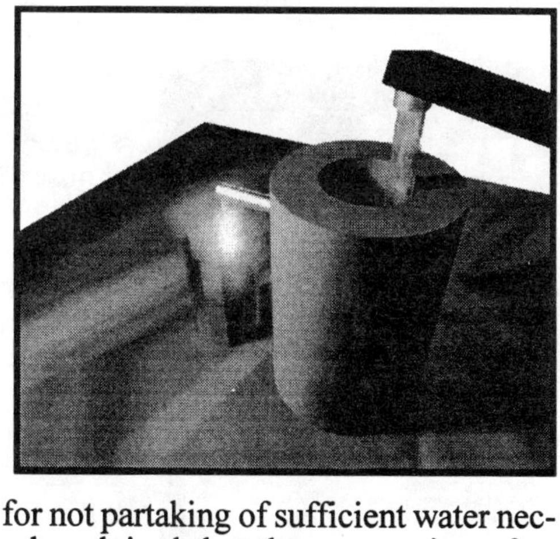

What about water in your diet? It is possible that many readers get a good portion of their water intake from juices and the water content in fresh vegetables and milk—about 85% water. Some will argue that the water sources are being polluted to the extent of their feeling better off not drinking the recommended 8 glasses per day.

If this is your excuse for not partaking of sufficient water necessary for bodily function, be advised that there are quite a few good water purification devices available today at reasonable costs. We have had one for many months and do agree that the water does have a much better taste when some of those chemicals are removed.

I am assuming that my body is also pleased with the results, though it has no method of communicating other than my continued good health.

Recently, emblazoned in the headlines of all national newspapers, was the report on cows' milk not being good for children. A report such as that can really "rock" a nation of Dr. Spock followers, until you study the background of the group publishing said report, the Physicians Committee for Responsible Medicine, a group which seeks to promote strict vegetarianism and animal rights.

They could have presented a much better argument for their case, had they studied (as I did) the research done by three authors, a medical doctor, a PhD and a nutritionist, in the book, *The X O Factor.*[22] These researchers concluded, with statistics, that the degeneration of arteries and increase in fat and cholesterol in the blood stream increased in great proportion with the homogenization of milk. Their research (to be brief) was based on the simple thesis that milk fat contains the enzyme xanthine oxidase (XO).

Homogenization breaks up the fat globules which enclose the XO (encapsulates) and protects some of the enzyme from being digested. As a result, the "escaping XO" is able to penetrate the intestinal wall into the circulatory system, where it is eventually deposited in the artery lining, causing atherosclerosis. However, the XO factor in milk is still not accepted as a real cause for the disease, according to other scientific reports. Naturally, the dairy industry didn't like that study any better than the recent explosion of newspaper headlines boldly stating that cows milk was not good for babies. I would say that that was quite understandable and imagine that a few thousand farmers didn't approve either.

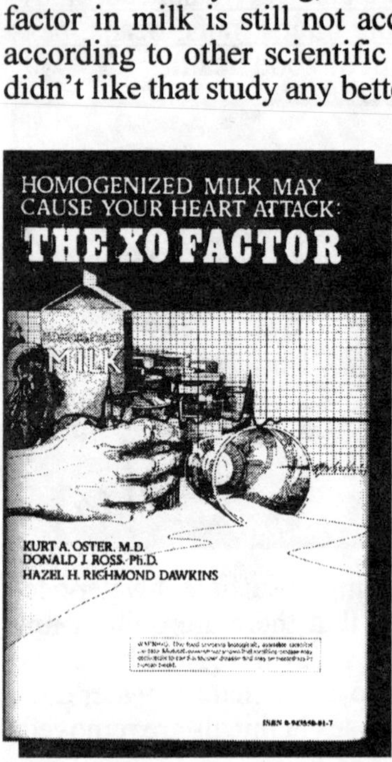

The mention of cows' milk reminds me of the Vermont country doctor, Dr. Jarvis, author of *Folk Medicine.*[23] He wrote extensively of the use of honey and apple cider vinegar to rejuvenate bodies deficient in potassium, even to the extent of having administered same to cows, at the request of local farmers, when their animals were hardly able to stand. The results were amazing and he went on to explain this combination being used for salmonella poisoning, early morning "blahs" after too much alcohol, chronic fatigue, dizziness and weight reduction. If you've never eaten cold baked beans (Boston-baked) with some apple cider vinegar thereon, you have missed a treat known only to old New Englanders such as myself!

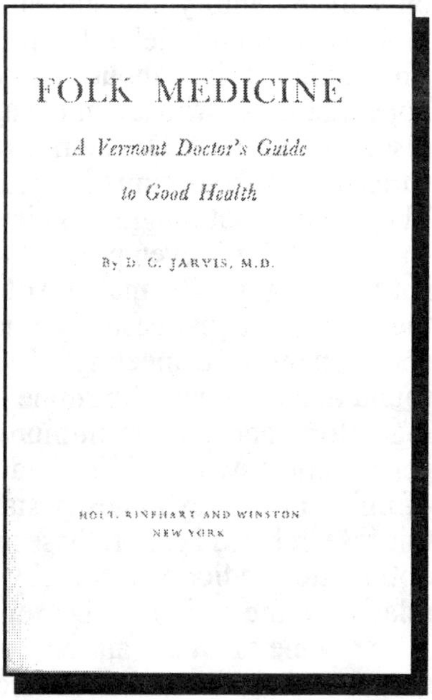
FOLK MEDICINE

A Vermont Doctor's Guide to Good Health

By D. C. JARVIS, M.D.

HOLT, RINEHART AND WINSTON
NEW YORK

Dr. Jarvis advised humans to "take a leaf out of the animals' book" —and—WALK more! Similar to animals roaming the fields in search of the greener grass, *always* on the other side of the fence! And, last, but not least, he wrote:

"*......the ideal of Vermont folk medicine is to condition the body in it's entirety so that disease will not attack it.*"

It seems that this good old country doctor was preaching the same thing mentioned within these pages a few times——***Preventive Medicine!***

Most of what we have been discussing herein relates to diet in one form or another, but, there are really no diets designed to ***prevent*** disease. I have presented a few theories and foods being used to stave off killing diseases, and, in many cases, remarkable results have been accomplished in alleviating the suffering from certain diseases or conditions. However, medical science is a long way from eliminating the illness and disease that plague humanity, and as progress is made relative to present illnesses, there will certainly be other forms coming into existence, such as the fury with which AIDS came upon society, practically unannounced until almost full-blown in nature. Agent Orange illness in Vietnam veterans and the unidentified disease now beginning to be evident among our Desert Storm veterans give us a picture of diseases never anticipated by medical reaearchers, a never-ending struggle for mankind and evidence that disease of some sort or another will always be with us.

In Chapter Thirteen, I wrote that when researchers announced the discovery of a potential cure for a certain disease or condition, future results were not as conclusive or did not prove the optimistic results anticipated. Recently, a new "trend" of optimum was voiced in a state meeting of the medical profession. The new "trend" is in the direction of "gene therapy" as a future cure or lifetime control for acquired diseases such as AIDS, cancer and diabetes, with a "one-shot" treatment. They were careful to relate that such research is only in the embryonic stages presently, and that one day we may look back and marvel at the primitiveness of present-day medicine. This author writes about this new research optimistically, though I hope that those who are in the age group primarily affected by these diseases such as AIDS, do not veer from their use of ***preventive*** measures due to the optimistic predictions that a cure is available soon. They should not magnify their expectations.

I don't even pretend to understand the extremely complex nature of the genetic makeup of the human immune virus as stated in the study, but just casually relate here the statements made in the above-mentioned meeting. Evidently, the research scientists have found that the human immune deficiency virus (HIV) contains self-regulators, and that an immune factor might allow our systems to permanently switch off the bad virus, or leave it in a less latent stage of infection. They honestly state that there is a long road ahead in this research and I exhort these medical researchers not to show overly optimistic predictions, thereby causing less ***prevention,*** especially relative to the serious AIDS epidemic facing us today.

None of what I am writing about herein is new, but may be to many readers. Some have read about same but have ignored it or "put it off until tomorrow." Therefore, once again, I implore you to follow these good recommended practices designed to ***prevent*** illness before it strikes!

To use a well-known tennis expression: ***"The Ball is in Your Court!" PREVENTIVE MEDICINE*** is not just a "catch phrase," and has been used repeatedly herein to emphasize the importance to your future well-being and health. ***Our*** health, and the savings in dollars from potential illness, depend completely and entirely upon each and every one of us. Follow a good nutritional diet to guarantee the health of our bodies now, and during those "golden years." Make them truly *golden* by embracing good nutritional habits now, for yourself and your children.

EPILOGUE

University of California at Berkeley Wellness Letter

THE NEWSLETTER OF NUTRITION, FITNESS, AND STRESS MANAGEMENT

Many times throughout this book I have recommended the *University of California at Berkeley Wellness Letter,©* "The newsletter of nutrition, fitness and stress management," to use the publication's masthead wording. While writing this book, issues of February 1993[30], Volume 9, Issue 5, and April 1995, Volume 11, Issue 6, prompts this epilogue because of the strong references to vitamins E and B, the real basis of the *Dr. Rinse Formula* booklet—the use of wheat germ, lecithin and oil or sunflower seeds. To quote the February 1993 issue directly........

"E: the evidence grows stronger

> "Vitamin E has been a celebrity among nutrients for a while now and in the past year research has been accumulating about this vitamin's role in protecting against some types of cancer as well as heart disease. If studies continue to back up these beneficial effects, even mainstream nutritionists may eventually advocate vitamin E for everybody.
>
> "What makes this vitamin so interesting is it's antioxidant properties—that is, it seems to gobble up free radicals (as do vitamin C and beta carotene). Free radicals are unstable molecules created by various normal chemical processes in the body. They can also be created by cosmic or solar radiation, cigarette smoke, and other environmental influences. Chemically incomplete, they "steal" particles from other molecules, creating more unstable compounds and thus setting off a chain reaction that can damage cells. This scenario may be one factor in the development of cancer, heart disease, and other chronic disorders. Of the hundreds of studies conducted worldwide on vitamin E, many have suggested that doses far above the recommended dietary allowance (RDA) may delay development of cataracts, bolster the immune system, reduce the risk of cancer and heart disease, prevent angina, combat toxins from cigarette smoke, treat Parkinson's disease, and have other beneficial effects. Unfortunately, some other vitamin E studies have not found any benefits, and others have been flawed or inconclusive. So the jury is still out, waiting for more evidence. Three recent studies

may help to tip the balance.

Oral cancer

"A major study published in May in the *American Journal of Epidemiology* found that people who took vitamin E supplements had half the risk of oral cancer compared to those who didn't take them. Vitamin E from foods, supplements of other individual vitamins, and multivitamins (which contain a relatively small amount of E) did not protect against oral cancer. Still most of those who took vitamin E took other supplements as well, so the rsearchers admitted that they couldn't rule out the possibility that it's a combination of vitamins that is protective."

"And it may also be that reduced risk is attributable to some hidden factor common to people who take vitamin pills, no matter how carefully the researchers statistically adjusted for known risk factors (such as tobacco and alcohol use). Another recent study published in *Nutrition and Cancer,* also found that vitamin E reduced the risk of oral as well as esophageal cancer."

Heart Benefits

"In November, at the annual scientific meeting of the American Heart Association, researchers from Harvard presented preliminary findings from two large studies that suggested that vitamin E supplements may reduce the risk of heart disease by one-quarter to one-half. One study looked at 87,000 female nurses, the other, 45,000 male professionals."

"Scientists theorize that vitamin E and other antioxidants decrease the oxidation of LDL ("bad") cholesterol—a process similar to butter going rancid—and thereby reduce plaque buildup in coronary arteries. The protective effect of vitamin E held after even adjusting for vitamin C and beta carotene intake. The reduced risk of heart disease was seen in people taking more that 100 International Units of E a day for at least two years, far more than you could get from food alone."

Should you or shouldn't you?

"It's important to remember that these Harvard studies, though exciting, have not yet been published, so the data have not been reviewed by other scientists. These reports may raise readers' hopes, as well as vitamin manufacturers' profits, but there are many potential problems with population studies that try to link individual nutrients with major diseases. We are anxious to see these studies, and are withholding final judgment until then. In addition, many other studies are underway, and it is hoped that these will verify the apparent benefits of vitamin E and help determine the dosage necessary to produce the protective effect. '*The evidence is very intriguing and promising, but I don't think it's good enough to support a widespread recommendation to take vitamin E,'* said Dr. Myer Stampfer, one of the Harvard researchers. **However, Dr. Stampfer noted that he himself, like many other researchers in this field, takes vitamin E capsules.** (Bold print is mine.)

Is the RDA enough?

"Many foods contain vitamin E. Vegetables oil (such as soybean, corn and sunflower) and products made from them, (margarine, for example) are the richest sources. Nuts and wheat germ are other good sources; green vegetables, beans and grain products are modest sources. Unless you eat these foods regularly, you may not be getting the daily RDA of vitamin E, which is 8 to 10 milligrams of alpha-tocopherol, the most potent form of vitamin E. That's equal to 12 to 15 International Units (IU), another measure of the vitamin—and about as much as in a cup of peanuts, 1/2 cup of wheat germ, or 3/4 stick of margarine."

"However, most studies that have found benefits from vitamin E have looked at much larger doses—generally 100 to 800 IU daily—than can be supplied by food. Even these doses of vitamin E appear to produce few side effects, though headaches and diarrhea have occasionally been reported. It's estimated that 4% of Americans now take vitamin E capsules, and more are likely to start. Reasonable supplementation—say, 100 IU daily—certainly won't do any harm. Keep in mind though, that the long-term effects of large doses of vitamin E supplements have not been studied in humans."

(Author's Note: Remember—before buying vitamin E capsules: ONE TABLESPOON OF LECITHIN IS EQUAL TO APPROXIMATELY 10 TO 12 CAPSULES!)

Following this publication on vitamin E, the *Wellness Letter* issue of April 1995 relates the discovery that Folacin or Folic Acid, the B vitamin abundant in leafy greens, seems to play a great role in preventing cervical cancer, and, that the content of vitamins B-6 and B-12 contained therein, may play a great role in preventing heart attacks.

As a result of these studies, this author continues to recommend your following the Dr. Rinse Formula booklet, incorporating into your diet the basic ingredients mentioned therein of **lecithin, wheat germ and oil or sunflower seeds** daily—PLUS—**brewer's yeast** which contains just about every element of the B vitamins.

There is a greater source of B12 in organ meats such as liver, etc., but they are very high in saturated fat and cholesterol. Dairy products and eggs are also high in B-12 which might be more acceptable in your diet than organ meats which do increase uric acid in the system. This acid is one of the recognized causes of gout, so you might want to follow the more attractive path in choosing your source of heavier concentration of B-12. Bear in mind that our bodies require very little vitamin B-12 and perhaps that is why Mother Nature was so sparing of it in heavy doses.

This *Wellness Letter* report on vitamin E follows my thought in a previous chapter about researchers using "disclaimers." They stated, "the jury is still out" relative to the long-term effects of large doses of Vitamin E in humans. I find it difficult to agree with that last sentence of this quote, however, due to the tremendous study and research done many years ago by the Dr's. Shute, Dr. Rinse and those other doctors who used heavy concentrations of vitamin E and lecithin in their treatments for cardiovascular and prostate conditions.

The December 1993 issue of the American Heart Association's journal *Circulation*, as reported in most national newspapers, stated that ***vitamin E had proved to be more potent than either vitamin C or beta carotene*** in preventing a first-step in the formation of the artery-clogging plaque that causes heart disease. This research was done at the University of Texas Southwestern Medical Center in Dallas, and one of the principal researchers labeled **vitamin E *the superior antioxidant*** after completion of the research.

For years I have been taking vitamin supplements whenever I was unable to have my usual breakfast consisting of items mentioned herein—-**wheat germ, brewer's yeast, lecithin, sunflower seed and whole grains.** I am especially pleased to see, however, that this quote from the *Wellness Letter*[30] certainly updates the information I have studied through the years relative to the value of Vitamin E in one's diet, and also reinforces what I have outlined in the first paragraph of Chapter Eight..........

Medical science is often finding studies that have previously shown the nutritional value of certain foods, "rediscovering" so-to-speak, medical knowledge previously attributed to foods such as

lecithin, studies reported upon years ago.

I have a Sagittarius calendar which one day gave this advice. Seems as though it might be good advice for all to follow everyday...

"TAKE THE HINT ABOUT NATURAL FOODS MORE SERIOUSLY. A WELL-BALANCED DIET, COUPLED WITH EMOTIONAL AND MENTAL EQUILIBRIUM, ACTS LIKE A SUPERCHARGED BATTERY."

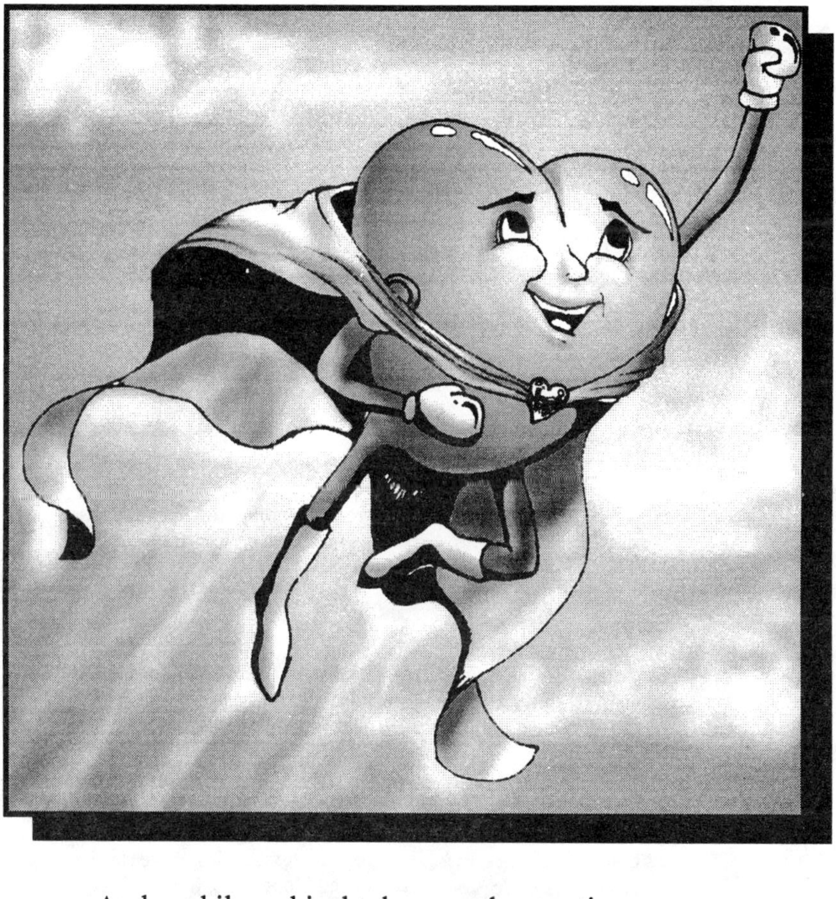

And a philosophical token worth repeating......
"Aging is not a disease, but a process you can deny!"

Good Health to all from this octogenarian!

THE FOLLOWING TABLES OF VITAMIN AND MINERAL SOURCES ARE PRESENTED TO OUTLINE THE MANY VITAMINS AND MINERALS PRESENT IN THE BASIC INGREDIENTS AS MENTIONED BY DR. RINSE IN HIS BOOK, AS WELL AS INTHE FOODS AS PRESENTED AND RECOMMENDED HEREIN AS POTENTIAL AIDS IN ALLEVIATING THE CONDITIONS WRITTEN ABOUT.

VITAMINS

A	Fish liver oils, dairy products, yellow, orange, and dark green leafy vegetables.	For healthy skin and mucous membranes, bone growth, reproduction, improves night vision, fights infection.
B	***Wheat germ, brewer's yeast, whole grains***, liver, oysters, soybeans ***(lecithin), lean meats, poultry, pork, fish, peanuts, black strap molasses, bran, brown rice.***	Complex vitamin B1 to B12. Nearly everyone needs it. Proper metabolism, skin disorders, anemia, stress affecting nerves and mental condition--You can't live without it!
C	Fresh fruits, citrus, tomatoes, melons, green vegetables, potatoes.	Antioxidant, prevents scurvy, wound healing, rough skin, loose teeth, fights effects of pollution in the body.
D	Fortified milk, egg yolks, liver, tuna, salmon. It's made on the skin in sunlight.	Promotes and is essential for normal strong bone growth and absorption of calcium.
E	***Wheat germ, soybean oil (lecithin), other vegetable oils, whole grain cereals, dried beans and legumes*** (all mentioned herein), peanuts, nuts, liver, green leafy vegetables.	Antioxidant of polyunsaturated fatty acids, essential to use of oxygen by muscles, increases life of red blood cells, inhibits blood clots (as outlined in lecithin section)

VITAMINS

BIOTIN	***Brewer's yeast, soybeans (lecithin), soybean flour,*** liver, brown rice, kidneys, egg yolks.	Formation of fatty acids and carbohydrates by metabolism.
FOLICIN (FOLIC ACID)	From B- vitamin family. ***Brewer's yeast, whole grains,*** liver, wheat bran, ***beans.***	Assists in forming body proteins. Important in synthesis of DNA, acts with B-12 in production of hemoglobin.
INOSITOL	***Brewer's yeast, whole grains,*** liver, citrus fruits.	Necessary for hair growth, brain cell formation, metabolism of fat.
K	Leafy green vegetables, cabbage family ***(sulphoraphane)***, milk, kelp, yogurt, egg yolks, polyunsaturate oils. (Made in the intestinal tract).	Essential for normal blood clotting, liver function and maintaining vitality and longevity.
PABA	Part of the B-complex. ***Wheat germ,*** liver, black strap molasses.	Necessary in body utilization of proteins, fats and carbohydrates, for hair pigmentation and formation of blood cells.
P (Bioflavinoids)	Part of the C-complex, buckwheat, citrus fruits, plums, grapes, cherries.	Works with and protects the strength of vitamin C.

MINERALS

CALCIUM	Milk, yogurt, cheese, ***whole grain cereals,*** sardines, salmon, shell fish, bone meal.	Bone formation and strength, blood clotting, nerve conduction, rythmic heart action.
CHROMIUM	***Whole grains, brewer's yeast***, meats, polyunsaturated oils, clams, ***broccoli, beans, peanuts.***	For glucose metabolism, synthesis of cholesterol and fatty acids, aids in action of insulin.
COPPER	Liver, ***whole grains, dried beans,*** raisins, almonds, leafy green vegetables.	Aids in formation of red blood cells, necessary for proper bone formation, helps to produce several respiratory enzymes
IRON	Liver, kidneys, red meat, egg yolks, peas, whole grains, brewers'yeast, fruits and vegetables.	For stress resistance, formation of hemoglobin, builds blood quality.
MAGNESIUM	***Whole grains,*** soybeans and soy products (lecithin), nuts, bananas, apricots, green vegetables.	Regulates normal heart beat, proper function of muscles and nerves, healthy maintainance of bones.
MANGANESE	Brewers's yeast, wheat germ, sunflower seeds, whole grain cereals, nuts, bone meal, egg yolks, cocoa.	For normal reproduction and cell function, necessary for protein, fat and carbohydrate production, and for skeletal developement.
IODINE	Iodized salt, seaweed, vegetable oils, dairy products, crops from iodine-rich soils (Example: Florida orange juice)	Necessary for function of thyroid gland and normal cell metabolism, also for healthy hair, skin and nails. Prevents goiter.

MINERALS

FLOURINE	Fish with bones (like sardines), tea, gelatin, fluorinated water.	Solid bone and tooth formation, prevents cavities.
PHOSPHORUS	***Whole grains,*** meats, eggs, poultry, dried fruits. In nearly all foods.	Bone growth, strengthens teeth, repair of cells, energy, metabolism, kidney function, proper skeletal growth.
POTASSIUM	***Whole grains, sunflower seeds***, tea, dried fruits, ***beans & peas,*** potatoes (with skin), coffee, yogurt, cocoa, bananas, meat, poultry, milk.	Necessary for muscle contraction, muscles and heart. Regulates blood pressure, proper maintenance of mineral and water balance in cells.
SELENIUM	***Wheat germ & germ of cereal grains***, bran, ***broccoli***, garlic, chicken, shell fish, red meat, onions and tomatoes.	Helps vitamin E fight cell damage acting as an antioxidant, aids in normal body growth and fertility.
SODIUM	Table salt, baking soda, prepared foods such as cheese, smoked meats, any salted snack.	Helps regulate water pressure and water balance.
ZINC	Brewer's yeast, wheat germ, milk, beans, eggs, liver, fish and meat.	Needed for cell division, healing and developement of new cells, aids enzymes in digestion and metabolism. Necessary for growth and normal functioning of the prostate gland.

BIBLIOGRAPHY

1. Davis, Adelle, *Let's Eat Right To Keep Fit,* Harcourt, Brace & Co., Inc., New York 1954
2. Orton, Vrest, *The Whole Grain Cookbook,* Farrar, Strauss & Young, Inc., New York 1951
3. Reader's Digest, *Eat Better Live Better,* Reader's Digest Association, New York/Montreal,1982
4. Wade, Carlson, *Lecithin,*
5. Rinse, Jacobus, *The Rinse Formula,* and,
6. Clark, Linda, *Know Your Nutrition, How to Improve Your Health,* Keats Publishing, Inc. New Caanan, CT. 1988, 1979, 1973, respectively
7. *The Wellness Letter,* University of California at Berkely
8. Rodale, J.I., *How To Eat For A Healthy Heart,* Rodale Books, Inc., Emmaus, PA 1954
9. Katahn, Martin, *The T-Factor Diet,* Bantam Books, New York 1989
10. Davis, Adelle, *Let's Get Well,* Harcourt, Brace & Co.1965
11. Harris, L.J., *The Book of Garlic,* * Harris Publishing Co., Berkeley, CA 1947-1984 ****Lovers of The Stinking Rose is a copyright of L.J.Harris and publishers of The Book of Garlic.***
12. *Organic Gardening Magazine,* Rodale Press, Dec. 1992
13. *The Washington Post,* Washington, DC April 22, 1984
14. Brown,T.McP & Scammell,H.,*The Road Back,*M.Evans & Co. New York 1988
15. *American Legion Magazine,* Indianapolis, IN Oct. 1992
16. Langer, MD, *Arthritis,* & Wade, C., *Arthritis, Nutrition, and Natural Therapy,* Keats Publishing Inc., New Canaan, CT
17. Miller, Mark, *Wine-a Gentleman's Game,* Harper, Row Publishers, New York 1984
18. Lucia,S.P,*Wine and Your Well-Being,*Popular Library,New York '54
19. Maury, E.A., *Wine Is The Best Medicine,* Universal Press Syndicate, Kansas City 1974
20. Rodale, J.I., *The Prostate,* Rodale Books, Emmaus, PA
21. Kenyon, Herbert, *The Prostate Gland,* Random House, NY, 1950
22. Oster, K., Ross, D.J., Richmond, H.H., *The X O Factor,* Park City Press, New York 1983
23. Jarvis, D.C.,*Folk Medicine,*Holt,Rinhart & Winston,NewYork 1958

24. Rinse, Jacobus, *The Absorption of Cholesterol, **1986***
Reynier, M.O. et al, Lipids 20, (3) 145, 1985
Small, D.M., J. Am. Oil Chem Soc. 45, (3), 108, 1968
Vandenheuvel, F.A., J. Am. Oil Chem Soc., 40, 464, 1963
Sycha, et al, See Pfeiffer, C.C., Health News & Review, 3/4, 11, 1986
Aldersberg, J., Mt. Sinia Hospital, 9, 995, 1943
Katz, S.S., J. Biological Chem. 256, 12275, 1981
Morrison, L.M., Geriatrics 13, 12, 1958
Koumans,A.K.J.&Wildschut,A.J.,Clinical Cardiology 8, 547, 1985
25. American Institute for Cancer Research, Spring 1992
26. Levy, Gail, American Health, New York, March 1986
27. Krech,Inez M., *Beans and Peas* Crown Publishers, New York 1981
28. Kreitzman, Sue, *Garlic,* Harmony Books, Crown Publishers, N Y
29. Oliver,Cap,MD,*Ongoing Treatment With Antibiotics,* T.McP Brown Institute, 5275 Lee Highway, Arlington, VA 22207, *The Scanner*, Winter 1992
30. Editors,*The Wellness Letter*,Univ. of California at Berkley, Feb. 1993
31. *The Wellness Encyclopedia of Food and Nutrition,* University of California at Berkeley 1992

OTHER PUBLICATIONS HELPFUL IN OBTAINING AND MAINTAINING HEALTH AND LONGEVITY

The Johns Hopkins Medical Letter, *Health After 50,* PO Box 420176, Palm Coast, FL 32142
The Vegetarian Gourmet, PO Box 7641, Riverton, NJ, 08077
The Walnut Acres Catalog, Walnut Acres, Penns Creek, PA
Choate, Judith, *The Bean Cookbook*, Simon and Schuster, New York, NY
American Institute Cancer Research, *Newsletter*, Washington, DC
Prevention Magazine c/o Rodale Press above.

To order additional copies of **My Lifetime Tidbits of Preventive Medicine**, complete the information below.

Ship to: (please print)

Name ______________________________

Address ______________________________

City, State, Zip ______________________________

Day phone ______________________________

_____ copies of ***My Lifetime*** @ $12.95 each $__________

Postage and handling @ $2.50 per book $ __________

Total amount enclosed $ __________

Make checks payable to ***Health -Mor Publishers***

Send to: P.O. Box 361
Georgetown, DE 19947

To order additional copies of **My Lifetime Tidbits of Preventive Medicine**, complete the information below.

Ship to: (please print)

Name ______________________________

Address ______________________________

City, State, Zip ______________________________

Day phone ______________________________

_____ copies of ***My Lifetime*** @ $12.95 each $__________

Postage and handling @ $2.50 per book $ __________

Total amount enclosed $ __________

Make checks payable to ***Health -Mor Publishers***

Send to: P.O. Box 361
Georgetown, DE 19947